PANDEMIC, GOVERNANCE AND COMMUNICATION

This book focuses on what is arguably the most devastating phenomenon in the history of modern civilization, the COVID-19 pandemic.

It shows how, on the one hand, the pandemic has exposed the deficiency of governments the world over in dealing with a major health crisis; and, on the other, it also reveals efforts by the ruling forces to enforce surveillance on people to disciplining them by maneuvering cutting-edge digital technology in the name of security and safety. Second, it explores how the mainstream versions of crisis communication and risk communication face huge challenges during a pandemic. Finally, it analyses how the pandemic propels an extraordinary expansion of infodemic — rapid spread of excessive quantities of misinformation and disinformation of the fake and false variety — and how social media in particular becomes its main tool in causing subversion of the prevalent information order.

Engaging, comprehensive and accessible, this book will be of immense importance to scholars and researchers of politics, especially governance and political communication, communication studies, and public health management. It will be vital for public policy professionals, experts in thinktanks, career bureaucrats, and non-governmental organizations.

Dipankar Sinha is Professor of Political Science and Director, Centre for Social Sciences and Humanities, University of Calcutta, India. He is also Honorary Associate of the Centre for Media History, Macquarie University. Sinha's research mainly focuses on communicative dialectics of governance and development in the post-globalization era. He has authored six books, co-authored four and co-edited two. He has also published widely in international and national journals and edited volumes.

Sinha's most recent books from Routledge are *The Information Game in Democracy* (2018) and *The Social Sciences in a Global Age: Decoding Knowledge Politics* (2021).

Routledge Series on the Humanities and the Social Sciences in a Post-COVID-19 World

The COVID-19 Pandemic has changed our lives economically, politically, socially, and emotionally.

The pandemic has impacted around the world in terms of health and wellbeing and brought into sharp focus fault lines and continuities in our lives and societies which are likely to outlive the pandemic. In this light, the humanities and the social sciences will have a crucial role to play as we reimagine and reshape everything we know in the post-pandemic years.

This Routledge series aims to bring forward cutting edge interdisciplinary research on various facets of politics, society, economy, environment, culture, psychology, and wellbeing in the post-COVID world. The books in this series will engage with a range of topical issues that have surfaced in the wake of the pandemic, and study how these emerging trends and critical developments are likely to impact the way in which humanities and social sciences are taught, researched and understood in the years to come.

Books in this series

Democracy and Public Policy in the Post-COVID-19 World
Choices and Outcomes
Edited by Rumki Basu

Pandemic, Governance and Communication
The Curious Case of COVID-19
Diparkar Sinha

Federalism and the Response to COVID-19
A Comparative Analysis
Edited by Rupak Chattopadhyay, Felix Knuepling, Diana Chebenova, Liam Whittington, Phillip Gonzalez

For more information about this series, please visit: https://www.routledge.com/Routledge-Series-on-the-Humanities-and-the-Social-Sciences-in-a-Post-COVID-19/book-series/HSSPCW

PANDEMIC, GOVERNANCE AND COMMUNICATION

The Curious Case of COVID-19

Dipankar Sinha

Routledge
Taylor & Francis Group
LONDON AND NEW YORK

Cover image: Getty Images

First published 2022
by Routledge
2 Park Square, Milton Park, Abingdon, Oxon OX14 4RN

and by Routledge
605 Third Avenue, New York, NY 10158

Routledge is an imprint of the Taylor & Francis Group, an informa business

British Library Cataloguing-in-Publication Data
A catalogue record for this book is available from the British Library

Library of Congress Cataloging-in-Publication Data
A catalog record has been requested for this book

ISBN: 978-1-032-11796-6 (hbk)
ISBN: 978-1-032-16180-8 (pbk)
ISBN: 978-1-003-24738-8 (ebk)

DOI: 10.4324/9781003247388

Typeset in Bembo
by SPi Technologies India Pvt Ltd (Straive)

Dedicated to
Frontline health workers and volunteers fighting the pandemic…
We survive 'cause you are here.

CONTENTS

PREFACE AND ACKNOWLEDGEMENTS

To deliberate on one of the most ubiquitous and mysterious phenomena ever faced by mankind let me begin with an apparently contradictory contention. The book was not needed to be written at all is as much true as the point that it was needed. The first contention has its rationale in the fact that we are in the midst of proliferating literature on the greatest pandemic in human history. The second contention has its logic in the fact that given the enigmatic nature of the pandemic there is always a scope to view and analyse it from varying vantage points. Let me assert that the proud human race never in its wildest imagination thought that a tiny pathogen called COVID-19 would devastate the world within a span of few weeks. Our supreme confidence that a pandemic may occur but we have made enough progress to counter it was demolished within days. The pandemic started playing havoc in a true global fashion, that too in different phases. People around the world were being hit in unusually hard ways— physically eliminated, economically shattered, socially distanced and culturally shocked.

The pandemic in the scheme of this book is a 'curious case' in a classical way because the phenomenon combines in all its subtlety and intricacy the elements of novelty, oddness, strangeness, unexpectedness and even the act of prying with an urge for inquisitiveness and exploration. However, this book has been written in a slow but steady pace. Let there be no doubt that the pandemic has led to an excessive growth of literature, many of which are basically based on a 'hurried glance' and too small snapshots of what is without doubt a phenomenon with exceptional magnitude and layers. Thus, one has to be a little slow in understanding the nature and impact of the pandemic, especially when one notices with much alarm that even a foremost social thinker of our times, Giorgio Agamben, faltered in understanding its enormity and complexity; it is to be discussed in detail in the book. The author's location in India, which faced an unimaginably tragic situation particularly during the second strain, a double mutation 'Indian' variant (technically called B.1.617) also required a patient understanding of the hard reality. No less so because living in Kolkata and in my home state of West Bengal, the reality was even harder because during the second wave every safety precaution was thrown to the wind by all political parties and by a large section of people, for whom the state assembly elections became more important than human lives. It was difficult to remain a 'detached observer' while being a witness to utter helplessness all around. Nor was it easy to concentrate amidst people literally struggling for breath and dying because of lack of minimum healthcare facilities. In direct contrast to the argument that governance should be scrutinised only during the 'normal' times and not during a grave crisis the prevailing situation strengthened my resolve to delve critically into the ins and outs of governance and its claims.

On another account, a slow process of thinking was possible because the coronavirus provided an unforeseen and unexpected 'study leave' by having the university closed for more than a year. Even if online classes were resumed after a point and online examinations were conducted the usual work pressure one faces being physically in the university was not there. The so-called new normal took its toll in robbing me of vibrant classroom interactions. However, some kind of consolation could be found in having found much greater scope of reading the huge literature on the pandemic, which ultimately resulted in this book. With burgeoning literature on COVID-19 pouring in from numerous sources one needed an uninterrupted long seclusion in the study to cope with it. The even more devastating second wave of the coronavirus transformed seclusion into solitude.

A distinct feature of the book is that that it is overwhelmingly based on the most recent publications. The Bibliography of the book reflects it. This was inevitable as the volume deals with a real-time phenomenon. There was also literally a struggle to cope with the continuously emerging literature dealing with every conceivable dimension and issue relating to the pandemic. Digital technology made it possible to be exposed to such literature, especially because physical access to libraries was closed for most of the time But at the same time, being inundated with articles, reports, blogs, documents, news items, interviews, memes, and with a limited number of books, it was quite a tedious task to pick up the relevant ones.

Writing a book on an ongoing event in such unsettling times would have been impossible without the exceptional support of family. So once again, special thanks to Mamoni, Saswati and Disha for letting me avoid most of the essential household duties. While Mamoni remained smilingly indulgent Saswati went through the pre-peer reviewed draft to make several important suggestions. Disha, a busy fintech content analyst herself, spared some time to explain a few intricate and tricky dimensions of virtual technology. The constant complaints about my seclusion by our two pets, good old Sparky and newcomer Ablu, had to be addressed by having them in the study. Let me mention that a number of former students and friends not only encouraged me to take up this venture but some of them supplied me with relevant material from other parts of India and from abroad. I thank them collectively.

This is my third successive book with Routledge, and I am indeed thankful to Aakash Chakrabarti, Senior Commissioning Editor, for untiringly keeping me on track. Frankly, this book would not have come out without him. I also thank Brinda Sen of Routledge for taking care of various technical requirements. The usual disclaimers apply.

Dipankar Sinha

INTRODUCTION

Rethinking pandemic governance

A random Google search with 'COVID pandemic' shows about 1,080,000,000,000 results in 0.86 seconds![1]

Within a short time, the pandemic has produced a mind-bogglingly vast array of literature in the natural and the social sciences. While non-scientific works have surged, the rigorous methodological compulsions and peer reviews have meant that scientific literature on the pandemic has been playing catch up. And not all of them are reliable or have come up with fruitful results. When the scientists, especially the virologists and epidemiologists, are struggling to find the modus operandi of the virus the economic, political, social and cultural manifestations of the pandemic are being analysed by others.

Perhaps the most serious questions in the non-scientific realm have been posed to the business of governing. Every government across the world faced the greatest challenge to its credibility, if not to its existence, with the pathogen wreaking havoc. While post-millennial governments know much more about managing epidemics and pandemics, they seem to have been a few steps behind throughout this pandemic. Public policies, which are in theory supposed to protect the interests of people and ensure their welfare, safety and security, were found wanting. There was no scope for course corrections midway, nor were there any best practices to fall back on. The motive force of public policy formulation and implementation in the current times, 'governance', including its high-tech, cutting-edge digital format, known as 'Governance 2.0', came under the scanner for generating surveillance, rather than welfare service. Its trump-card of efficiency, more concerned with citizen vigilantism than anything else, faced severe criticism for the failure to protect the lives of crisis-torn people. In the process it was proved beyond doubt that effective governing primarily rests on 'physicality', the human factor.

States around the world were in large measure found to be unprepared to face the mounting challenges. A major problem was the excessive faith placed in technocratic

DOI: 10.4324/9781003247388-1

solutions. In India, for instance, as the ruling political leadership and a section of bureaucracy boasted about employing digital means to combat of COVID-19, the virus hit back with a devastating second wave. With people dead and traumatised, both physically and psychologically, promises of welfare, safety and security seemed like empty rhetoric. It was only the pro-active role of the frontline health workers and volunteers, who made valiant efforts at the grassroots level to check the progress of the pandemic.

More generally, the pandemic, by the first quarter of 2021, has caused more than three million deaths. It has zealously infected people, snatched lives, affected countries irrespective of their developed/underdeveloped, east/west or north/south status. To add, the visible costs of the pandemic have been staggering, but its invisible costs make it the costliest pandemic, both in human and economic terms.

Countries that were perceived as 'knowledge hubs', widely admired for their national healthcare facilities, faltered. That Britain with a strong national healthcare system would become the epicentre of the second phase of the pandemic tells its own tale. Such is the power of the virus that even populist world leaders, who promised to deliver a solution 'very soon', were embarrassed and questioned. In many cases, to hide their failure in governing States sought to curtail the freedom of expression of disenchanted people. Leave aside the authoritarian countries, even democracies, such as the USA and India, have been accused of fomenting mis/disinformation around the pandemic.

A report of the Freedom House (Repucci and Slipowitz, 2020), a democracy watchdog in the US, sharply criticises the handling of the pandemic by the Trump administration. Unsurprisingly, though, it specially refers (ibid., p. 10) to the former US President's press conferences and social media posts which 'repeatedly downplayed the severity of the coronavirus, attacked state governors from the opposition Democratic Party for imposing social distancing measures, promoted unproven treatments and false health statistics, asserted that the pathogen would soon disappear, and pushed for restrictions to be lifted even as the contagion spread, among other harmful statements.'

It may be pointed out that in Trump's defeat in the presidential election in November 2020, his pandemic policy, or perhaps more appropriately its absence, played a certain role. In the same report, India has figured (ibid., p. 4) under 'categories of abuse' like restrictions on media, restrictions on protest, detention or arrest of dissenters, and police violence. The report found that the pandemic has intensified a crisis for democracy around the world; and since the outbreak democracy and human rights indices have dropped in as many as 80 countries. It also notes that governments have responded to the crisis by abusing power, silencing their critics and weakening or shuttering important institutions, thereby often undermining the very systems of accountability needed to protect public health in such crisis times.

However, confusion abounds. With numerous analysts coming up with observations and suggestions, there seems to be a 'tower of babel' insofar as our understanding of the COVID-19 pandemic is concerned. This is not to say that there are no informed and reasoned analyses available, but the fact remains that such analyses are outnumbered and overwhelmed by the instantaneously produced literature. This book seeks to confront this situation with a specific take-off point; it advances the argument that there is a need for according urgent attention to the known–unknown dialectics in order to develop ontological, epistemological and methodological perspectives on the pandemic. The dialectics not only concern the 'new normal' but it will be an integral part of what is being termed as the 'next normal'.

Pandemics and epidemics have traditionally provoked exceptionally creative minds to come up with new ideas. It certainly set up the stage for Leonardo da Vinci, the legendary Renaissance polymath, during the bubonic plague in Milan in 1484–1485, which eliminated 50,000 people – one third of the city's population. He had stayed back in the city and watched it unfold. He went on to create a new design for the city which till date is much admired for combining aesthetics and efficiency in reconceptualising and restructuring urban space – an essential component of what in today's world is termed as urban governance. How would da Vinci have reacted to the coronavirus pandemic, which is infinitely bigger than what he had confronted? Would he have been able to come up with a new blueprint of governance globally, and not just for a city? Hypothetical questions, but they are worth pondering.

Centuries later, in a different part of the world, another polymath invested his genius, energy, time and funds in confronting malaria and visualising an alternative form of 'governing' epidemics in Bengal in India in the early 1920s. He was the poet-philosopher, Rabindranath Tagore. He had witnessed the ravaging impact of malaria, plague, cholera, tuberculosis and smallpox and the mismanagement that accompanied the efforts to control them. Its impression not only found a place in some of his novels, stories, essays, poems and letters but also spilled over to his activism. He made Santiniketan (the abode of peace), where he had established a university, the prime location for this endeavour. He focused his efforts on collecting funds from local and foreign friends and organising human resources to build anti-malaria health cooperative societies. His zeal for acquiring grassroots level experience in this regard is important to mention here because he provided important insights into the act of governing during the epidemic times. He was not content in blaming the imperial rule for the calamity. On the contrary, he placed much emphasis on the creation of community awareness and engagement for local-rural reconstruction, based on generation of 'self-power' as a way of countering the calamitous situations.

Which also brings us to the main concern of this book: governance.

Governance involves deep and often not-so-deep structures, numerous modes of behaviour, countless human affiliations, and, no less, deceptive maze of human ties. Governance here is perceived as a product of a specific historical juncture with certain delineated attributes, which will be discussed in detail in Chapter 1. The issue is not that of circulating a ready manual for preparedness in times of crisis. It is a much larger issue, as I shall argue, of being ready to face the unknown and not being obsessed with the known.

Governance by itself is a contested concept. When governance experts appreciate its academic travel on a 'bumpy road from enfant terrible to a relatively mature paradigm' (Sørensen and Torfing, 2018:1) they allude to its controversial impulse and its yet-to-attain maturity status. One agrees with them that governance is here to stay, but when it comes to their assertion (Sørensen and Torfing, 2018:7) that the paradigm is robust enough to 'analyse, inform and guide concrete governance practices', one has to be a little more cautious as an analyst. It is not being argued that any paradigm, especially with such power and reach, should be free from contestations, or that it should attain maturity. However, it is a fact that in the face of the pandemic the multisectoral approach to problem-solving and crisis management of governance have exposed its weaknesses. Even the steadfast advocates of governance are desperate to justify it in such turbulent times. Judging by the trends in what I shall describe as the governance-in-practice during coronavirus times it may be helpful to use the analogy of 'stop motion' to explain how it seems to be functioning. In this technique, widely used in animation films, objects are physically manipulated in small increments between individually photographed frames and when the frames are sequentially played back, they appear to exhibit independent motion or change. In a similar vein, failure of governance can be attributed to, among other factors, similar incremental changes in the business of governance (and governance is indeed business now!) are falsely projected as change for the better. If one remembers this analogy, it will be easier to understand my take on governance in the book – how the governance-in-thought periodically comes out with recommended frames of change, and how on the contrary the governance-in-practice, in its zeal to present a too neat picture, moves with chimera of motion to deny such changes.

The COVID-19 catastrophe has created certain practices of the unconventional kind. To provide an instance, community engagement, which became an important strategy during the pandemic and has been extensively discussed in Chapter 4 of the book, acquired a performative aspect. In India, during the first wave of the pandemic, responding to the call of the Prime Minister, Narendra Modi, people switched off electricity for a stipulated period of nine minutes and lit candles, earthen lamps, torches and cell phones accompanied by full-throated chants of 'Go Corona, Go'. On other occasions, again at the behest of the Prime Minister, people would also indulge in 'balcony performances' by clanging utensils to articulate their appreciation of frontline COVID workers like doctors, nurses, healthcare workers, sweepers and so forth. Overenthusiastic citizens took out processions bursting crackers in expressing their disgust against the virus and promising to free Mother India from its scourge. Some would go at length to put forth 'scientific' reasons to justify these acts, with explanations such as the capacity of sound and light waves to minimise the impact of coronavirus. In their zeal to support the government's interventions to counter the virus many would go beyond the stipulated nine minutes and those participating in the street processions would defy another stipulated norm, social distancing. These citizen-centric 'performances' should not be taken lightly nor be they seen only in terms of their immediate entertainment value. They are also to be interpreted as significant instances of political communication with persuasion and manoeuvring public opinion at the core to legitimate governance actions and hide inactions and failed actions by the same stroke.

Though analysis of public policy communication has been described (Sinha, 2021:47–59) as a 'nearly lost theme' in policy analysis the fact is communication remains the lynchpin of governance – both as a solution and as a problem. The pandemic and the state of the world in the days of global interconnectivity reminds one of Paul Virilio's chilling narrative in *City of Panic* (2005), written in the background of intersections of speed, space and terror. It depicts how cities like Paris are targeted by the 'weapons of mass communication', the harbingers of the new technological revolution. As a result, cities are transformed into epicentres of anxiety, devastation, disaster, distrust, emergency, fear, paranoia and vulnerability. In a way Paris in such narrative is a metaphor for the world. Much is being written on the ways and means of administering the pandemic but comparatively little on its communicative aspects and dynamics. Those who treat communication as a secondary process and pay only concessionary attention to it tend to miss both the foundation and the modus operandi of governing, governmentality and not the least for our purpose here, *governancing* (I shall throughout use the unconventional term, courtesy of Levy-Faur, 2012:9). The trouble is that when communication is accorded some attention in the study of governance it is mostly seen as an ancillary process of digitalisation – at best as e-governance. The other kind of literature on governance, mainly in the form of reports by the activists, has lot of focus on communication but it rests on a markedly managerial approach, which perceives the instrumental power of communication to penetrate 'good governance' messages among the 'target groups'.

There are, however, few prominent exceptions to the general trend. How deep and extensive communication has become is evident in Negri's analysis in *The Politics of Subversion: A Manifesto for the Twenty-First Century* (1989). Though he has a different locus and context, and the understanding the 'social' character of the labour-production dynamics of the contemporary times, the way he posits the importance of communication is worth noting in our context. One of his most notable comments (ibid.: 48) is that in contemporary society communication is simultaneously the connective element as well as the point from which to exercise control. It is so because, as he argues, it counterposes the equality of community to that of money, utopia to cynicism and productive cooperation to capitalist control. Having pointed out that 'social' production finds its exclusive centre in communication, in the processes of information and in the spheres of communicative structure, Negri adds that under the domination of capital, however, the mode in which communication functions and takes shape is simultaneously a mode of expropriation. What he also adds (ibid., p. 58) subsequently has much greater implications to enhance our understanding of the communicative impulse of governance, the way it is being presented in this book. He refers to the aim at gaining control over communication (that is, to desire its reappropriation) to influence in a direct way the social relations of production and exploitation. It is on the new organization of communication that the determinations of exploitation are based.

There is also another academic strand, as found in *Governance as Social and Political Communication* (Bang, 2003), which decisively connects governance with communication. One of the core points in the approach, which is more optimistic than the one adopted in this book, is the concern (ibid.: 1–2) with the 'steering' and the practice of freedom in a 'high modern' world with increasingly complex, dynamic and differentiated everyday life. Bang himself refers to Janet Newman's *Modernizing Governance* (2001) and asserts (Bang, 2003:5) that the 'governance shifts' identified by Newman in terms of ten major propositions 'involve communicative turn in policy analysis'. The ten propositions are as follows:

(i) A move away from hierarchy and competition as alternative models for delivering services towards networks and partnerships traversing the public, private and voluntary sectors.
(ii) A recognition of the blurring of boundaries and responsibilities for tackling social and economic issues.
(iii) The recognition and incorporation of policy networks into the process of governing.
(iv) The replacement of traditional models of command and control by `governing at a distance'.
(v) The development of more reflexive and responsive policy tools.
(vi) The role of government shifting to a focus on providing leadership, building partnerships, steering and coordinating, and providing system-wide integration and regulation.
(vii) The emergence of 'negotiated self-governance' in communities, cities and regions, based on new practices of coordinating activities through networks and partnerships.
(viii) The opening-up of decision-making to greater participation by the public.
(ix) Innovations in democratic practice as a response to the problem of the complexity and fragmentation of authority, and the challenges this presents to traditional democratic models.
(x) A broadening of focus by government beyond institutional concerns to encompass the involvement of civil society in the process of governance.

Newman's propositions are based on her contention (Newman, 2001, p. 39) that governance cannot be viewed as a free-floating phenomenon, understood simply through the lens of universal trends such as globalisation or growing social complexity. She insists that the approach to governance that can be found at a specific time in a specific place has to be understood in the context of particular political conjunctures. These propositions will come up in one way or the other in this book but what is to be noted here is that except on one occasion (ibid: 29) of linking communication with power in the discourse theory Newman did not devote much space to the communicative dimensions in her analysis of governance.

In this book, however, communication is the key to contextualising governance during the pandemic and among pandemic publics. Here, communication – conceived as a process of creation, generation and neutralisation of meanings – is foundationally social but it has an ingrained political attribute in the sense that it involves many processes of inclusion and exclusion based on various hierarchies. Communication is connected to the act of governing, governability or governance as a political process in the broader public realm in which the political regimes negotiate their acts with the people. It is also concerned with the governed, made up of numerous messages, signals and symbols of the ruled, and in this domain too it is socially grounded and politically dynamic insofar as it relates to power equations of numerous kinds. In my explanatory framework the 'political' and the 'social' in communication are too intimately connected existentially through countless strands to detach them at ease and at will.

I stick to this framework though I know for sure that a clearer connection would have been ideal and analytically more convenient; at least it would have opened up fewer questions. Then again, simpler analyses, howsoever convenient, are not something social scientists are fated to live with. Take the case of communication itself. If the analysis here relies on its linear interpretation it would be impossible to show how during the pandemic, despite the best of efforts on the part of ruling establishments around the world to control and enforce top-down information flow, there would be sources of 'leakage', defiance and subversion. In other words, this would have made the pandemic a much less complicated phenomenon than it actually turned out to be.

One major point in the debate on the COVID-19 pandemic is up to what point it is indeed an 'equaliser'. There is a dominant perception that it spares none and cuts across all barriers. It is true that the virus spreads across all forms of boundaries – social, political and economic. However, there is a parallel argument being floated that its transmission rate among the 'lower classes' is less. In India, for instance, there is a discussion in the public domain that the virus has mostly spared beggars on the street who are most vulnerable to infections of all kinds because of their insecure life, and for whom 'social distancing' is not only an alien concept but also an unaffordable practice. On a lighter note, a spoof on YouTube channel has become extremely popular, in which an American coronavirus scolds its subordinate counterpart in Bangladesh for under-performance and inactivity, citing the failure to fulfil the target of infected people.[2] In response, the coronavirus from Bangladesh pleads helplessness and explains because that the country with people habituated to poor living and health conditions has made it immensely difficult to break the immune system. At the end, the American coronavirus admits the difficulties encountered by the virus in Bangladesh, and in a sobering tone appeals to it to try its best to wreak havoc. However, the class bias in a completely different way becomes not only evident but grave when it comes to the post-infection stage – in the treatment of the poor infected patients in the abysmally inadequate and discriminatory healthcare sector in developing countries. Then again, the bias is a result not of the modus operandi of the virus, but of the skewed nature of human intervention which in this case is part and parcel of 'governance'.

The book

Chapter 1 focuses on the enigmatic core of the unprecedented pandemic. It argues that the pandemic's relations with us are paradoxical: it is impossible to live with it as much as it is impossible to live without it. The pandemic, to reaffirm the subtitle of this book, is indeed a 'curious case', with ingrained novelty and intricacy, and its fair share of secrets, mysteries, concealments and silence zones. What is noteworthy is that all these attributes are not only relatable to the occurrence of the pandemic; they also engulf the process of exploration of its antidotes, the vaccines, to the point of raising doubts about their efficacy. In this backdrop the *known–unknown* dialectics is identified throughout the volume as the constitutive core of the pandemic dynamics and of numerous forces negotiating and/or countering it. In the process the chapter puts forth the provocative argument that the 'unknown' is bound to have an indelible mark in understanding and analysing the pandemic. It is indelible because the chance of 'knowing everything' about the pandemic is very slim. Relevant ideas and activities of the transnational organisations, especially the WHO (World Health Organization), various national and international agencies and governments from around the world are discussed along with the most recent writings on the nature of the pandemic by leading social theorists and scientists to show the imprint of the known–unknown dialectics. In the analysis communication is accorded a significant status, not as an end in itself, but as an essential mediating force for sustaining the dominant form of (pandemic) governance and the counter-search for alternative modes. The chapter also brings into the limelight the complex intersections, tensions and fault lines in the struggle to come to terms with the 'unknown', and refers to the downsides of the temptation to obstinately stick to the 'known known'. The discussion then moves to the interpretation of the pandemic as a flexi-modern development, with the social theory of late modernity set in the background. Here again, the purpose is to reinforce the main line of argument that an understanding of the pandemic to a great extent rests on approaching the 'uncertainty' phenomenon and that the rigid and monochromatic interpretations of the same are bound to be misleading and self-defeating.

The next chapter traces the roots of the now-dominant notion of 'governance'. It does so by identifying it as a particular brand of governing, emerging from the neoliberal project in circulation since the 1990s. The basic argument in the chapter is that notwithstanding the periodic theoretical endeavours to reframe and refine the idea of governance the 'actually existing governance' – governance-as-it-is /governance-in-practice, characterised by strategic, codified, technocratic and decontextualised knowledge – has grossly underperformed during the pandemic times. Highlighting 'good governance', the most publicised and the most aggressive form of governing in contemporary times, the analysis shows how its foundational pillars – accountability, transparency, participation, responsiveness and efficiency – are found to be deficient in times of crisis.

In a nuanced assessment, the chapter also refers to the failure of the counterforces seeking to come up with viable alternative/s to (good) governance. The deficient performance of (good) governance is attributed to its 'one-size-fits-all' orientation which seeks to discipline knowledge by stifling the exploration of the 'unknown' with excessive claims over the 'known'. The communicative dialectics of governing, especially the importance of governance communication, is also addressed with due importance. Thus, it critiques the dominant mode of communication by noting the steady weakening of the human-sourced *connections* by the digital network-sourced *connectivity*. Keeping the pandemic governance model in the forefront there is deeper discussion, with references to some leading scholars of governance, of a break between the change-orientation in theory building in governance and the status quoist orientation of its practitioners. The analysis arrives at a major contention that in the act of governing it is essential to realise that knowledge and ignorance are inseparable, in both existential and ontological terms. The chapter also takes up the vital issue of migrant workforce as a case of poor governance. Using documentary evidence it shows how governance under-performance forces them to bear the major brunt of the COVID-19 pandemic. The chapter, however, concludes that considering the dearth of effective alternative governing approach/es neoliberal governance will continue to rule devising new and updated strategies.

The third chapter has an extensive treatment of the major mode of *governancing*, sourced from biopolitics and biopower. The discussion has a specific focus on the communicative dynamics of the biopolitical mode – in the instrumentalisation of life and objectification of personhood through substantive and symbolic messages. The fundamental argument that runs through the chapter is that the mode is being manoeuvred during the pandemic times by the ruling regimes around the world, with the goal of controlling the body, mind and conduct of populations. It is also argued that beyond such overdrive there lies an 'offense is the best defence' strategy, meant to hide the abject failure in governance in crisis times. Beginning with Michel Foucault's pioneering ideas on biopolitics and governmentality but going beyond to address more contemporary and deeper studies on the theme by later scholars the analysis also highlights the innovative and subtler ways of relegating the 'unknown' to the background by the powers that be. It also refers to the twin processes of the 'biologisation of the digital' and the 'digitalisation of biology' to explain how they contribute to the millennial biopolitical instrumentality in two major ways:

i) Shaping the emerging force of (bio)informational capitalism.
ii) Forging biocitizenship – the creation of 'obedient' subjects by injecting a deep sense of insecurity, which also leads to popular demand for more vigorous practices of restrictive rules and norms.

Explaining why the pandemic is not just a medical crisis but a social, political and ideological crisis of mammoth proportions the concerned issues are sought to be interpreted in the lens of the neoliberalism-capitalism, its strategisation of public health in particular.

Chapter 4 seeks to assess the growing body of the community engagement literature – with special emphasis on communicative dynamics – in the light of the pandemic outbreak. Noting that the ideas about 'community engagement' have surfaced and intensified since the 1990s, coinciding with the growing hegemony of the governance paradigm, the discussion concentrates on the 'engagement/disengagement paradox' to observe that the COVID-19 pandemic has vehemently reinforced the stiff challenge of negotiating and/or reconciling 'engagement with 'distancing'. In emphasising the simultaneity of engagement and disengagement the chapter also scrutinises the contours of crisis communication and risk communication, the vital thematic sources of exploring and managing outbreaks and catastrophes. Analysing the existing literature on (community) engagement communication the chapter identifies the fundamental problems in an overwhelming concern with 'action plan' orientation in the case of the crisis communication, and with the 'toolkit' approach in the case of risk communication. In the process it also finds their converging point in linear interpretations of information flow and in ready-made solutions to problems and challenges. The multiperspectival analysis also shows how, despite having recognised 'community' as a locus of shared interest and environment, and crisis and risk as the essential items to negotiate the pandemic situation, there is an attempt to marginalise the 'political' dimension. It is argued that such 'apolitical' mission results in skewed communicative dynamics breeding inequitable and non-participatory power relations in the name of wellbeing of people.

The final chapter concentrates on one of the most significant developments in the millennial information and communication order – the infodemic and its subversive capacity. Infodemic is the rapid spread of excessive quantity of mis/disinformation, which threatens to make the classical tenets of ideal communication – reliability, credibility, trust and relevance – irrelevant and meaningful solutions to problems more and more elusive. Its implications for governing in crisis times is explained in terms of (virtual) platform politics of social networking sites and social media. There is specific focus on the role of the tech giants which exert overwhelming control over the information flows to establish oligopolistic control. The analysis combines the key findings of academic research, advisories of transnational organisations (including the WHO) and policy documents of various civil society organisations to reveal how coronavirus becomes a hyper-active source of numerous mis/disinformation, with far-reaching economic, commercial, political, social and cultural impacts and cross-boundary impact. The chapter then focuses on some possible countermeasures against infodemic but goes on to make another provocative argument that both social media and information technology, two prime tools of informational capitalism, by their very constitutive logics retain the possibility of manoeuvring infodemic in their own interest, at least for the time being.

The ensuing discussion in the book reveals how multifarious and ultra-dynamic the process of 'rethinking' has to be when it comes to dealing with pandemic governance. In promoting new horizons, issues and events and at the same time manoeuvring the existing ones, the process maximises complexity and challenge for any analyst. As if it acquires a 'never ending' form, with little scope for complacency and guaranteed solutions.

Notes

1 As of 26 June 2021.
2 Baul TV Bangla: 'করোনা ভাইরাস বাংলাদেশে এসে পারিসানিতে পড়ে গেছে', ('Having reached Bangladesh coronavirus faces stress') https://www.youtube.com/watch?v=i_w5q8Jd0d8, accessed on 28 June 2021.

1

UN/KNOWN

Negotiating COVID-19 in highly uncertain times

Introduction

To repeat what has been asserted earlier, it is impossible to live with COVID-19 and it is impossible to live without it. The paradoxical statement best sums up the mysterious pandemic and the highly unsettling times sourced from coronavirus. Having its supposed origin in Wuhan, China, in late December 2019, the pandemic struck the world with lightning speed since January 2020 – a year which will be remembered by all for a long time. The Novel Coronavirus (SARS-CoV2), a deadly pathogen, penetrated body and soul of people around the world in a way no one could ever imagine. Even keeping in mind Albert Camus' placement of pandemic and war side by side in terms of their shock value in his classic *The Plague* (2010 [1946]) one can argue that in some ways even the most devastating wars pale in comparison to this pandemic. In course of time, COVID-19 may lose its momentum but as a catastrophe of never-before magnitude it has left an indelible influence on us – on our life, livelihood and living. Those who dare to announce that 'it's over' prove themselves, especially with the subsequent arrival of the more-severe 'second strain', to be either ignorant or prophets of false claims. The crux of the matter is that a virus, which is almost weightless and invisible, has not only been able to cause a screeching halt to the so-called march of human civilisation but it has also been able to change gear of human evolvement forever.

There is not a single inch of the existential reality, which remains unaffected by the virus. Human body might have been its prime target, but it is not the only one as society, economy, polity and culture have been 'infected' in their entirety. There is much truth in the observation (Lupton and Willis, 2021:5) that the crisis it brought 'is a complex and ever-thickening entanglement of people with other living things, place, space, objects, time, discourse and culture'. At the same time, as already mentioned, the virus has displayed a great show of fairness in infecting people from all walks of life – making no distinction, not even between the powerful and powerless.

DOI: 10.4324/9781003247388-2

It truly became global, arguably the most global phenomenon ever, by transcending all physical boundaries and defying all restrictive rules of cross-country movement. Yet, the most distinctive attribute of COVID-19 is its enigmatic core. Even with so much attention piled on it much of it remains is yet to be known. Let it be asserted that the post-COVID world will continue to bear this imprint and there is little scope to think otherwise. In foreseeable future there is no escape from the effects of the virus even if physically its presence is reduced. The following observation (Kindig et al., 2020) provides a glimpse of the predicament with which we are fated to live:

> We will go outside. The pandemic will fade, for now. The future will come, imperfect but alive. But what will be left in the sand when this tide has ebbed? We can hope it might be robust mutual aid networks, a renewed commitment to the commons, a fighting movement for Medicare for All. Even should this be true, there will also be mass unemployment, hundreds of thousands of deaths, gutted social infrastructures, global supply chains on the verge of collapse, and a devastated planet.

To reiterate, the COVID-19 pandemic is a 'curious case' par excellence, worthy of further exploration – but without the guarantee that everything about it would be exposed.

Approaching the pandemic analytically involves a rider of foundational import. The rider concerns the dialectics of the known and the unknown. I shall argue that the dialectics will continue for such a long time that we shall hardly ever reach a stage in which all that is unknown about it will be known. In more precise terms, the dialectics will not reach an end any time soon. COVID-19 has led to a burgeoning literature, some of which will be used in the book. A substantial part of the literature reveals an overt or covert claim: that the impending task is to make everything transparent about the modus operandi of the virus. There is no doubt that unravelling the virus that has vastly changed our ways of living is important and it is not something that is to be done at a later stage. But the problem with an obsessive search for transparency is that it moves away from the sustained complexity of the known-unknown dialectics. Let me unfold the point gradually in the following discussion.

A pandemic extraordinaire

The greatest challenge of COVID-19, the most dreaded type in the coronavirus family, lies in its propensity to remain shrouded in mystery. Nobody has any clear idea about it. The only consensus is that it is the cause of a crisis which is much more than epidemic. On 11 March 2020, the WHO formally announced that the virus has led to a pandemic. In its definition a pandemic is 'the worldwide spread of a new disease' (WHO Website 1). There is no universally accepted definition of pandemic and this remains a contentious point in various debates (Honingsborn 2009:1939; Morens et al., 2009:1,018–1,021; Qui et al., 2016–2017:1–11). For instance, one major point of discussion is that if at all and to what extent a level of explosive transmissibility and severity of infection are required to declare a pandemic. Various issues, such as, severity, geographical extension, locus of movement, high attack rates, explosiveness, infectiousness, minimal population immunity, contagiousness, severity and novelty/newness are mutually linked in describing growth of disease as pandemic. The technical explanations of these features are best left to clinical, diagnostic and biomedical specialists, especially to virologists and epidemiologists. But the point of consensus even amidst the debate is that pandemic is a much larger and much more extensive form of epidemic. The magnitude and complexity of the pandemic comes out well in the following comment (Peters, 2020:1):

> The philosophy of pandemic is truly a philosophy for all peoples. It reflects not only the human significance of pestilence and plague, or the rise of modern viruses like COVID-19 that show the transition across species but also themes of individual/community – self-interest and collective responsibility, the sacrifice of first-contact health workers, and all of those who in the ethic of the other, provide a level of care in a neoliberal age less bound by duty or ethos of service and more by market values.

Debates continue on the question of according 'pandemic status' to historic outbreaks like Bubonic plague and Spanish flu, and to the more frequent ones like Tuberculosis, Malaria and Cholera, and to even more recent types like H1N1 outbreak, Ebola plague, cholera, SARS, MERS, H7N9, Ebola, Zika and HIV/AIDS. With the passing of time a disease accorded the pandemic status may be demoted to the status of an epidemic. A good example is Malaria, which used to pervade the world as a pandemic earlier but now is mainly confined to tropical countries, and thus being described as epidemic. But as hinted above, there can be no doubt that COVID-19 not only fits the bill to be a perfect pandemic but also occupies the top rank in the list of pandemics witnessed so far by humanity. By its sheer reach, magnitude and gravity – with millions infected and more than a million dying – it lays to rest the debate that the pandemic discourse is overhyped. The dominant variants of the second strain of the virus, unleashing the COVID Pandemic 2.0 since December 2020, with faster rate of transmission, and the simultaneous rise of vaccine hesitancy, vaccine anxiety and vaccine scepticism, reveal the herculean task of administering the pandemic. There are instances of trouble from unexpected sources as well, which only complicate the situation. Thus, for instance, in India at the very beginning of 2021 the two major vaccine providers were involved in a bitter war of words when one accused the other of not only inventing something which is only 'as safe as water'.

The point to be noted here is that perhaps the only settled fact about the virus is its ability to generate a disease of pandemic proportions. Everything else is either being still explored or is based on facts which are either contested or unverified or remains simply unknown. This is what brings us to consider the known-unknown dialectics. Then again, COVID-19 cannot claim to be the first pandemic to develop a mysterious character. Nor is it to be the last one. In this context one can refer to McMillen (2016:9), who informs that even knowledge about plague, recognised widely as the first pandemic in human history, is incomplete. He writes:

> What we do not know about the first pandemic overshadows what we do. This may change as more sophisticated tools of analysis become available. Careful reading of textual sources can get us only so far. Historians will need to draw from disciplines, such as, zoology, archaeology, and molecular biology if the mysteries of the first pandemic are ever to be revealed.

Leading scholars of pandemics like McMillen (2016:120) and Honingsbom (2019) prophesise with much confidence that pandemics are not going away and there are more to come. As Honingsbom notes (2019:266) after reviewing a century of outbreaks, 'the only thing that is certain is that there will be new plagues and new pandemics. It is not a question of if, we are told, but when. Pestilences may be unpredictable, but we should expect them to recur'. He also goes a step ahead of Camus in stating that the attempt to anticipate disaster also creates new distortions and introduces new uncertainties. Coronavirus has proved both of them right to an alarming extent. This also makes the dialectics more relevant, if not unnerving.

The consensus about the coronavirus disease being a pandemic does not solve the problem for social scientists. It is because they are primarily concerned with pandemic narratives. COVID-19 has been the most important example till date of numerous narratives of varying shades and shapes, which are in social circulation. The scientific studies of the pandemics are being given much importance. But studying pandemic narratives is important for several other reasons: they are important means of communication – between governments (within and beyond the borders of a country), between governments and people (in terms of both government-to-people and people-to-government interfaces) and not the least, among people themselves. In this complicated triad there are also transnational actors, such as, the WHO, and intermediary agencies like media, political parties, interest groups, non-governmental organisations (NGOs), civil society organisations (CSOs) and community-based organisations (CBOs). Davis and Lohm (2020:22) aggressively advocate the case for pandemic narratives in these words: 'Pandemics make for good stories, so good that there is an argument that they are implicated in the form and force of narrative itself, particularly those that help to bring into being collective life.' Two important points for the purpose of understanding the approach in this book are to be found in their analysis (p. 188): first, they relate pandemic storytelling across public life in dialogue to the narratives on the enactment of expert advice. They call it a dual approach. Second, and this point is even more important for the subsequent discussion in this book, they do not remain content by just pointing out that narratives do not simply mediate pandemic knowledge. In scrutinising health issues in a deeper vein they note that the associated narratives are not very far removed from the now discredited notions of linear, hypodermic communication.

Both points have vital importance in understanding the complexities of dialectics to be discussed below and throughout the book. The governance and communicative dynamics related to the COVID-19 pandemic assume much greater complexity because it demands a far more flexible approach. Such approach collapses, to the extent possible, the hitherto rigid divide of clinical and non-clinical realms and calls for synergy of every segment, professional and otherwise, of society to confront the crisis. The biomedical and epidemiological experts, along with public health physicians, infectious disease experts, nurses and health workers, are bound to be in the forefront of the battle against the pandemic. However, any effort to undermine or denigrate the role of other professionals, including the social scientists, would be self-defeating. Even if they may not have an immediate role in combating the pandemic social scientific analyses assume lot of importance in developing a certain kind of knowledge about the pandemic.

From one angle the pandemic of our concern is a social phenomenon of mammoth kind. It has affected societies as a whole and not in bits and pieces. In infecting individuals with astonishing speed it has threatened health and wellbeing of communities. It has generated not just fear but sheer panic irrespective of race, nationality, ethnicity, colour, religion and so forth. How complicated the pandemic politics is may be proved by the responses it elicits. In an interesting theoretical venture the phenomenon of fear, as articulated during the pandemic, is being interpreted as a 'motivating dynamics in politics' (Degerman et al., 2020). Citing the constructive role of fear in effecting compliance with public health restrictions during the pandemic such stance finds the positive perception of fear in the writings of Hobbes and Judith Skhlar more relevant in the current context than the denigrating role assigned to fear by scholars like Martha Nussbaum, Zygmunt Bauman, Hannah Arendt and Sara Ahmed. In another instance it has been argued that what may apparently seem to be a highly altruistic motive may turn out to be simply a case of self-interest. Žižek, in a dramatically titled book, *Pandemic! COVID-19 Shakes the World* (2020a), mentions that the reason behind the Israel government offering help to the Palestinians to combat coronavirus was not out of humanitarian motive but because of the fear of the Israelis being infected by the Arabs. The pandemic politics, it needs to be added, has other important dimensions too, one of which is medical diplomacy. Thus, India sent hydroxychloroquine, a preventive medicine for COVID-19, to 55 countries, apparently as a humanitarian gesture. In the case of US, however, the then President Trump, true to his style of functioning, had issued a direct threat to India to provide substantial quantity of the medicine or face the unpleasant consequences. In the case of others, including the Islamic states like UAE and Pakistan, India 'volunteered' to do indulge in the humanitarian act with latent diplomatic manoeuvring. In January 2021, India also sent large quantity of vaccines to her immediate neighbours and also to some Arab countries and Brazil. This led to the boastful description of India as the 'pharmacy of the world' by the Indian Prime Minister. However, he was later severely criticised by many for not leaving adequate stock of vaccines to save his own people from the scourge of the second strain. At this point, let me also note that being what it is COVID-19 will attract numerous 'backend' thinkers and analysts with social bent of mind. The pandemic is a social phenomenon too. An analysts of pandemic sociology pertinently points out (Dingwall et al., 2013:168) that there is a lack of basic understanding that medicine and biomedical science are no less social institutions. It is because they are carried out in social organisations by people who are socially recognised as competent practitioners within a division of labour; that they are delivered through other organisations and through social interactions with innumerable partners. It is also further explained that problems come to medicine and biomedical science along the socially constructed pathways and are delivered into the world by other pathways. This is why knowledge or technology transfer is a social process. It is asserted on behalf of the social that an exclusive focus on medicine and biomedical science only creates incomplete and truncated narratives of how societies identify new diseases, how they respond, and what the consequences might be. Another sociological view (al-Basam, 2020) on the biopolitical implications COVID-19 employs three types of psycho-social criteria: (a) epidemic of fear; (b) epidemic of stigmatisation and moralisation; and (c) epidemic of action and adaptive reaction. From yet another vantage point Aaltola (quoted by Carney and Bennett, 2014:136) views disease as a 'socially interpreted physical and physiological process' fundamentally shaped by prevailing political culture and practices. In this way, he adds, pandemic scares can be identified as polysemous, yet forceful, idioms of distress and anxiety. Chapter 4 of the book will take up this issue in the specific context of biopolitical measures adopted by the rulers for intensified regimentation of populations in pandemic times.

Notwithstanding such observations by a section of their peers the social scientists, let us admit, have long been indifferent to the study of virus. The contention remains true despite a few brilliant studies on pandemics in recent times, some of which are being referred in different parts of the book. It may be hypothesised that such lag in social sciences largely results from an underlying idea that 'invisible' viruses are not an integral part of the society, or that even if they are their duration is too minimal to merit any extensive and dedicated discussion. Caliskan and MacKenzie (2020) argue that an overly anthropocentric focus in social sciences leads to the neglect of pathogens. It is this 'eclipsed vision', they assert, which left social scientists unprepared in the current global crisis. They observe in an introspective vein:

> We, social scientists, have failed to see how viruses and people are related. Anything non-human escapes our vision; we filter it out. Such gross negligence makes it impossible for us to prepare for non-human actors with which we live, and that act like us. Viruses and people have many similarities. Much as humans do with the Earth, coronavirus damages the host in which it lives… Both humans and viruses live to exist.

One cannot agree more with their suggestion that there is a need to rewrite social science books with a focus on human and non-human interactions and their implications for society. At one level social scientists can help the policymakers in particular by providing cues about differential perceptions, attitudes and behavioural responses in 'heterogeneous' society by investigating variables like age, gender, socio-economic status/class. Within the broader social, cultural political and economic parameters, with vital ethical and normative issues, including the question of social exclusion/inclusion vis-à-vis resource allocation at the centre stage, clues about health seeking behaviour of various social strata, nature of regulation of livelihoods, creation and generation of panic and stigma, role of rumour and mis/disinformation and the role of media can be provided. The accumulated empirical evidence can not only aid the practical act of governing, of public health in particular, but it can also create a good amount of credible and relevant theoretical literature to enhance greater understanding of the impact of the elusive virus and the resultant pandemic. The pace and the traffic one finds in the COVID-related social science literature at present induces one to declare that the virus will surely be the most analysed one in social sciences in the years to come.

Then again, the task by any means will not be easy in terms of revelation, especially if there is a tendency to produce instant solutions. It will not be easy for social scientists because natural scientists themselves, who are supposed to provide leads about the nature and activity of coronavirus are yet to make confident claims that they have definite clues about it. Social scientists also need to take guard against the apparently authoritative but basically superficial claims of politicians around the world that scientists are soon going to unravel the mystery of the virus. Cees Hamelink (2020) in this context clarifies that it is better to keep in mind that science and political policy making live in two different worlds, and that governments and scientific research are 'not happy partners' as science avoids equivocalness and rests on complexity and differentiation, and politics on the other hand thrives on consensus building. He is of the opinion that the fundamental problem lies in the different approaches of the two domains: politicians look for quick and unambiguous answers while science is better at asking questions than providing answers. In the specific case of the COVID-19 crisis, he adds, science is 'speechless' – not only because it has no answers to the secrets of the virus but also to the questions about the economic, psychological, educational and cultural issues arising as a result of the measures to contain the pandemic. Warning against the possible complacency of social scientists about credible theory-building Hamelink notes how in science a combination of theoretical constructions are constantly bombarded with fundamentally new insights, with the outcome that even in the core of science every theory can be refuted. He then uses traditional metaphors (to be discussed in detail in the next section) in summing up his contentions: politicians want to be sure that all swans are white, underlining predictability, while science persistently searches for the black swan, emphasising the unpredictable part.

Unpleasant it may sound, much of the literature emerging in the wake of the pandemic seems to have been driven by knee-jerk reactions. The reflex of posting instant response to what is often described as the most mysterious pandemic did not spare even a veteran philosopher like Giorgio Agamben (2020a) who, in a brief article published in late February this year, equated it with normal flus and criticised in strongest possible terms the 'frenetic, irrational and entirely unfounded emergency measures' adopted by the Italian government for 'mild, moderate symptoms'. In assessing the 'real situation' he also underestimated the power of coronavirus by describing the disease as 'alleged epidemic' and confidently claimed that a miniscule four per cent of the population in Italy would require intensive therapy. Agamben also accused the media of being in league with governmental authorities in spreading collective panic with the virus as an 'ideal pretext'. He would find in the 'disproportionate' preventive measures of authorities a clear provocation of an 'authentic state of exception' and an effort to establish it as a 'normal paradigm' with serious limitations on movement and suspension of daily life. He identified and opposed the following major decrees on the ground that they restrict freedom: a) prohibition against any individuals leaving the affected municipality or area; b) prohibition against anyone from outside accessing the affected municipality or area; c) suspension of events or initiatives of any nature and of any form of gatherings in public or private places, including those of a cultural, recreational, sporting and religious nature, including enclosed spaces if they are open to the public; d) closure of kindergartens, childcare services and schools of all levels, as well as the attendance of school, higher education activities and professional courses, except for distance learning; e) closure of public of museums and other cultural institutions and spaces; f) suspension of all educational trips both in Italy and abroad; g) suspension of all public examination procedures and all activities of public offices, without prejudice to the provision of essential and public utility services; and h) enforcement of quarantine measures and active surveillance of individuals who have had close contacts with confirmed cases of infection.Agamben does not have an iota of doubt that 'in a perverse vicious circle, the limitations of freedom imposed by governments are accepted in the name of a desire for safety that was created by the same governments that are now intervening to satisfy it'. His contentions instantly provoked fellow philosopher, Jean-Luc Nancy, to respond in much critical terms. The very next day, in an article on 'Viral Exception', Nancy (2020) pointed to Agamben's failure to note that the exception is indeed becoming the rule in a world where technical interconnections of all kinds are reaching a hitherto unknown intensity which is growing at the same rate as the population. Nancy also warned that we must be careful not to hit the wrong target as living in an era of pandemic 'viral exception' – biological, computer-scientific and cultural – governments are 'nothing more than grim executioners'. In Nancy's view, taking it out on governments, as does Agamben, seems more like a diversionary manoeuvre than a political reflection. Agamben is not the lone figure in the initial act of misreading and undermining the gamut of the COVID-19 pandemic. However, what is also important is that the instance of Agamben-Nancy debate reveals that there is little scope to take things for granted and to indulge in instant observations insofar as the pandemic is concerned.

Known-unknown dialectics

In the light of the preceding discussion let us agree that COVID-19 as the mega-unknown element hides more than it reveals. Accordingly, the pandemic it creates is not only based on the known-unknown dialectics at present but it may remain so forever. To reiterate, there may never come a day when everything about it will be crystal clear, with nothing left to speculation. Even with the best of scientific efforts, including the most sincere and sustained biomedical and epidemiological initiatives, there will be many scientific and extra-scientific variables at play to keep a large portion of it unknown.

The inescapable role of the 'unknown' in a study of the H1N1 'swine flu' in 2009 has led to an interesting conceptualisation by Mansnerus (2010) of the 'silence of evidence'. She draws attention, on the basis of pandemic risk assessment of the flu, to the non-accumulation a robust body of evidence for decision-making and the presence of 'uncertainties' not just in epidemiological studies but also in historical and archaeological studies. The yet to be discovered/interpreted/found elements or factors are termed as 'silent evidence'. It is pointed out that the definition carries a tension within itself. Apart from the usual questions like who are at risk and what will happen globally, she mentions (p. 3) that the tension arises out of some such questions: What actually remains unknown? How is this 'lack of knowledge' conceptualised? In what sense could unknowing be seen as silence of evidence in the decision-making processes? Whose evidence remains silent, whose evidence speak for themselves? What then are the implications of 'silent evidence' for pandemic influenza risk assessment? Mansnerus contends that the urgency and unpredictability present in the course of a pandemic require that decision-making accommodates unknown factors, perhaps by standardising them over time. It is because, she explains, despite various attempts to standardise factual knowledge there remains a tension that manifests itself at a level of uncertainty, no less important being the fact that evidence itself is 'prone to contestations'. Describing uncertainty and unpredictability as part of a larger 'erosion crisis' one scholar (Spurk, 2020) comments:

> These experiences are part of...the erosion of the established world sliding into the unknown. Nothing is certain, reliable, or predictable anymore, as if we were standing on a sand dune that is slipping away under our feet. Certainly, our feet are on the ground, but the sand is moving; no one knows the reason, the direction, the extent or the duration of the shift. In such a situation of uncertainty and helplessness, resignation and fatalism tend to prevent us from taking responsibility for ourselves, and efforts to merely adapt to the new circumstances are widespread.

He links the erosion crisis to the reproduction of globalised capitalism on the ground that it demands the (self-)mobilisation of the subject to deal individually with this situation in order to find their place in society. He also adds that it contributes to the fear of globalisation and experiences of powerlessness that can lead to populism: an 'escape from freedom' into submission to a leader, a nation, a set of traditions. These points will be extensively deliberated in subsequent chapters. At this juncture let me note that this pandemic is not the first to have triggered off the dialectics being referred here. The interplay of the 'known' and the 'unknown' has a fairly long and rich history in any case and it has come under the philosophical scanner in many interesting ways.

To provide a brief reference to its recent history, Donald Rumsfeld, former US President George W. Bush's Secretary of Defense, made a statement in a press conference on 12 February 2002, in the context of US's confrontation with Iraq. The statement which provoked both admiration and sarcasm became known as the Rumsfeld's wisdom (Oxford Reference, 2017):

> As we know, there are known knowns; there are things we know we know. We also know there are known unknowns; that is to say we know there are some things we do not know. But there are also unknown unknowns – the ones we don't know we don't know.'

It generated some degree of admiration because of its epistemic value. Thus, Michael Shermer (2005), the author of *Science Friction*, finds in the statement a cue about science being sourced from the known meeting the unknown. Žižek (2006:137) on the contrary takes a sarcastic jibe at Rumsfeld for dabbling in 'amateur philosophising' and failing to include a fourth category, the 'unknown knowns', the things we do not know that we know. The fourth one, as Žižek reminds us, is linked to the Freudian unconscious, the 'knowledge which doesn't know itself'. The academic debate may go on but what is more important in the discussion here is that the pandemic and various responses to it have resurrected the known-unknown dialectics in a major way. Rumsfeld as a 'non-academic practitioner' has more than served our purpose by bringing the known-unknown back to limelight and it is because he did so thinkers like Žižek could make it a reference point and enrich our understanding of the utility of the framework in analysing public debates on a phenomenon of huge public importance. Arguing that apart from true or false solutions there are also false questions Žižek notes (p. 142) that the task is not to provide answers or solutions, but to submit to critical analysis the questions themselves, to make us see how the very way we perceive a problem is an obstacle to its solution. In this explanation he underlines the role of 'unknown knowns', which as silent presuppositions we are not aware of, determine our acts – 'mystifying our perception of the situation instead of allowing us to think it'.

A number of metaphors, analytically rejuvenated earlier in the context of financial management and/or disorder, become worthy of attention in further understanding of the exceedingly complex dialectics vis-à-vis the COVID-19 pandemic. Swans in particular, the black, white and lately the green variety,[1] have gained popularity in this regard. Let me begin with the metaphor of Black Swan. It is an old invention, conceptually refined by Nassim Nicholas Taleb, which has found a new lease of life during the pandemic. Taleb, an academic and by his own description a 'self-styled practitioner of uncertainty' and 'empirical sceptic', upholds (Taleb, 2010:17) that a small number of Black Swans 'explain almost everything in our world' – from events and issues in the public realm to personal lives. Black Swans are rarely found and seen. But it effectively reveals why we impulsively fall prey to the temptation of simplification, narration and categorisation, not being able to take into consideration what we don't know. The metaphor carries three main attributes: First, the rearity: it is an *outlier* as it lies outside the realm of regular expectations, because nothing in the past can convincingly point to its possibility. Second, its extreme impact. Third, the retrospective (though not prospective) predictability: in spite of its outlier status, human nature makes us concoct explanations for its occurrence *after* the fact, making it explainable and predictable. The formulation is of much importance for our discussion because of Taleb's claim that logic makes what we don't know far more relevant than what we do know. He also asks readers to consider that many Black Swans can be 'caused and exacerbated *by their being unexpected*' (p. 19). One of his most significant statements (p. 20) is as follows:

> What is surprising is not the magnitude of our forecast errors, but our absence of awareness of it. This is all the more worrisome when we engage in deadly conflicts: wars are fundamentally unpredictable (and we do not know it). Owing to this misunderstanding of the causal chains between policy and actions, we can easily trigger Black Swans thanks to aggressive ignorance – like a child playing with a chemistry kit.

Taleb also takes on the we-know-the-best attitude of experts by noting that our inability to predict in environments subjected to the Black Swan, coupled with a general lack of the awareness of this state of affairs, means that certain professionals, while believing they are experts, are in fact not so. He explains (p. 20) how the 'experts' cast influence on people by arguing that based on their empirical record they do not know more about their subject matter than the general population, but they are much better at narrating – or, worse, at smoking us with complicated mathematical models. In an earlier book in which Black Swan found its place for the first time Taleb (2001) had explained what he calls the *triplet of opacity*. They are: i) the illusion of understanding, or how everyone thinks he knows what is going on in a world that is more complicated (or random) than they realise; ii) the retrospective distortion, or how we can assess matters only after the fact, as if they were in a rear-view mirror (history seems clearer and more organised in history books than in empirical reality); and iii) the overvaluation of factual information and the handicap of authoritative and learned people, particularly when they indulge in 'Platonicy', the tendency to use concepts and models which obscure reality and generate wrong impressions of it. It may be added that in a television interview in late March 2020, Taleb controversially describes the coronavirus pandemic as a White Swan and asserts that it was 'preventable'.

For a deeper understanding of the dialectics one can mention yet another metaphor, Grey Rhino, which has a complementary connect with Black Swan. Grey Rhino, sourced from a Wikipedia reference but theorised by Michele Wucker

(2016) in *The Gray Rhino: How to Recognize and Act on the Obvious Dangers We Ignore*, refers to a highly likely yet ignored threat. In this case the colour game is trickier. As Wucker explains, there are black rhinos and white rhinos, but the black ones are not actually black, and the white ones are not actually white. They're all grey, but the catch is that nobody generally talks about the most obvious point – that all rhinos are grey. The metaphor indicates that by not paying enough attention to the big obvious problems confronting us we only make ourselves vulnerable to misdirected polities which are otherwise avoidable. In the case of COVID-19 we have let loose the Grey Rhino a number of times: primarily in harbouring the belief that we have made enough 'progress' to save ourselves from any such pandemic and also, as is evident from some examples cited in this section, some brilliant thinkers severely underestimating the power of the pandemic and its strike capability. This is how Wucker rationalises (2016:xvi) her favourite metaphor:

The Gray Rhino is a road map for recognising and learning from the times we have failed to get out of the way of a clear and present danger, and applying those lessons to the decisions we make when we have a chance not only to prevent a crisis, reducing human and financial costs, but also to create opportunities. Getting out of the way of a Grey Rhino can mean many things. It can mean embracing a threat and turning it into an opportunity. Yet it also can mean avoiding damage or, at least, minimising it. Acting in time can make a situation dramatically better. It can also merely keep a crisis from deteriorating, like the stimulus plans that followed the 2008 financial crash. Often enough, so much damage is done that things can never get back to normal, but if the damage done is the least of many worse outcomes it's still a significant improvement. Avoiding being trampled rarely, if ever, means keeping the status quo.

In an interview Wucker (in Jaye, 2017) posits the Grey Rhino metaphor against the Elephant in the Room metaphor to further strengthen the case for the former. She states:

> The elephant in the room is, by definition, something that nobody talks about, and nobody does anything about. The elephant in the room says to you, "Saying and doing nothing is normal." The gray rhino says, "No, it's not normal. You do have a choice. It's not inevitable that I'm going to trample you." Gray rhinos are things people are talking about, but not doing anything about.

On an empirical level the confusing signals emitted by front ranking actors like the WHO seem to be confirming the relevance of the Black Swan and the Grey Rhino in varying degrees. The WHO is now a beleaguered agency, not only because of its alleged China-friendly acts but also because of some shifting, conflicting and confusing recommendations. One of its worst and most impractical decisions, presumably done under political pressure from China, was to exclude from the WHO orbit a country like Taiwan which achieved much success in effectively calibrating governmental and the non-governmental sectors in tackling the pandemic. On the issue of the WHO letting loose a confusing scenario let me supply a rough list of the shifting observations and prescriptions since January, 2020: there is little to worry about coronavirus; it is basically zoonotic, which means that it normally resides in animals but can on occasions infect humans; it does not harbour human-to-human transmission; there is no need to cancel the Chinese new year celebrations; international flights from and to China need not be restricted. Then the gear is shifted and such recommendations follow: it is a global pandemic; no need to wear masks unless in confined places; everybody should wear masks outside home; the virus is not air borne and is only caused by droplets; the virus may be air borne; do not take hydroxychloroquine as a preventive; hydroxychloroquine as a preventive is effective and need to be taken; there is hardly any possibility of the spread of infection from asymptomatic cases; asymptomatic cases can spread the disease.

The WHO waited till 11 March 2020, to declare the COVID-19 phenomenon a pandemic and 'enemy of humanity', only after more than 1,20,000 cases were registered. This is despite the fact that after initial information blockade China had informed the UN agency on 31 December 2019, about a 'pneumonia' spreading in Wuhan, often called the home of the virus. But the WHO is not alone in contributing to such perplexing situation. As the apex healthcare agency of the world it certainly needed to be more prompt in actions, but the stupor was also evident in some countries, such as Switzerland, which is known for having robust public health systems. These countries were caught completely off guard when the pandemic struck. Even the former US President Trump, who was the most vociferous critic of the WHO and its Director General, Tedros Adhanom Ghebreyesus, displayed a totally lackadaisical attitude with the misplaced priority of saving the economy, which resulted in huge number of infected cases (including himself) and deaths. One cannot but remember his over-confident twit, all in caps – 'We cannot let the cure be worse than the problem itself' – urging the nation to be promptly back in business. Britain followed the US but there again the disease did not spare Prime Minister, Boris Johnson, from being infected and hospitalised. Brazil's President Jair Bolsonaro met the same fate after defying and denigrating restrictive measures on the pretext of putting the economy back on wheels. France had displayed an initial hesitance in undertaking preventive measures, leading to a marked decline in the popularity of President Macron. Nor can one ignore the failure of an otherwise highly disciplined country like Sweden, which was treated as an outcast by the neighbouring Scandinavian countries for not following the lockdown measures and being a laggard in ensuring herd immunity. In yet another instance, the EU has been criticised for its exceedingly slow response in alerting Italy about the fast spread of the virus in that country. The instances show that there was a problem, either in having 'adequate knowledge' of the pandemic or in 'having too little'. Both the varieties incidentally are linked.

Enough hints have already been dropped in the discussion here to assert that from the very beginning COVID-19 was fated to remain mysterious. There is a widespread impression in the world that the virus had escaped from a laboratory in Wuhan, China, but some scientists have expressed doubts about this proposition (Cyranoski, 2020). The governments and media around the world have acted in tandem to blame China for unwillingly or willingly let loose the virus and various motives have been attributed for this act. President Trump had led the blame game with aggressive allegations against China but there are a host of world leaders who agree though in a more sober tone that the outbreak was planned by the Chinese leadership. China has been accused of stifling the voice of Chinese scientists and doctors who sought to raise an alarm about the virus. The main whistle-blower, Li Wenliang, an ophthalmologist working at Wuhan Central Hospital, had sent a warning to fellow doctors on 30 December 2019. He was diagnosed with coronavirus on 30 January 2020, and died in February. Social media, especially Weibo, the popular Chinese microblogging site, was being extensively used by the Chinese people after his warning became public, but soon it faced strict official censorship. The western media, even those which were not on friendly terms with Trump, took on China with much vigour. Politicians were not far behind in China baiting. In one such case (Heydarian, 2020), presumably emboldened by Trump, Eric Schmitt, the attorney general of the state of Missouri in US, sought a Supreme Court ruling on the legality of a lawsuit against Chinese authorities, not just against the Chinese government but also against the Chinese Communist Party and senior Chinese officials for having 'deceived the public, suppressed crucial information, arrested whistle-blowers, denied human-to-human transmission in the face of mounting evidence, destroyed critical medical research, permitted millions of people to be exposed to the virus, and even hoarded personal protective equipment'. A civil society group followed suit accusing China of resorting to 'international terrorism' by unleashing the pandemic on perceived enemies. It is a different question whether in the US judicial system the legality of such cases could be entertained but they do indicate an anti-China hysteria revolving around the pandemic. However, there is another side of the story as well. In a parallel move China has resorted to soft power diplomacy in publicising her success in containing the pandemic. There is a report (Hernández, 2020) that the Chinese leadership and strategic thinkers have adopted a strategy to 'utilise' the pandemic situation to make a show of efficiency of China in containing the virus in comparison with the failure of countries pursuing 'democratic governance'. There is also the counter-opinion (Green and Medeiros, 2020) that this effort to gain credibility by China has few takers among the world leaders.

As expected, China vehemently opposes the allegations and seeks to disown any responsibility, even going to the extent of accusing the US of unleashing the virus. The visit of the WHO team of experts in the country in the last week of February 2020, did not bring any transparency about China's role in making the virus global. A report (Report 1, 2020) of the WHO-China Joint Mission contains many points about the nature of the virus and preventive measures but it is silent about the Chinese role, except for the acknowledgement (p. 4) that the first coronavirus patient was found in Wuhan. This is despite the very first item (p. 3) in the Goals and Objectives section of the report being the enhancement of understanding of the evolving COVID-19 outbreak in China. The report rather commends (p. 17) China's 'bold approach' and more surprisingly, 'exceptional coverage', and also cites strict 'adherence' and 'commitment' to the containment measures at governmental (national, regional and local), community, family and individual levels. Such blanket appreciation of the Chinese initiatives obviously raised eyebrows.

Amidst numerous events and processes the virus continued to unravel its mysterious nature, with leisurely pace. The common symptoms – fever, tiredness, dry cough, sore throat, nasal congestion, runny nose and diarrhoea – were subsequently supplemented by loss of taste and nausea. The new items lead the experts to declare that the excessive reliance on earlier symptoms was 'misleading'. There is either complete lack of knowledge or at least much uncertainty about a wide range of issues (Cereceda, 2020a): whether the virus is laboratory-born, when would effective vaccine against the virus will be invented and made available in market, how many people can be infected by an infected person, whether only droplets are the only means of infection, to what extent masks are effective to prevent infection, what kind of climate facilitate or hinder the growth of virus, whether the virus will surely lead to successive outbreaks after a phase of reduction, whether infection can recur in the same person, what exact role does co-morbidity play in an infected person, and last but not the least, whether the world will ever be free of the virus. Many of the unknown elements and entities, strengthened further with limited testing and inadequate accounts from most countries, substantiate the claim that the knowledgeable claims about the modus operandi of the virus is to be fraught with utmost caution. One such claim by some Italian scientists revealed that it is not caused by virus but by bacteria responsible for clotting blood and hindering transport of oxygen throughput the body. The fact-check (The Logical Indian, 2020), however, dismissed it. Graham Medley (2020), an expert in pandemic modelling, candidly mentions in a BBC interview that anyone who predicts what will happen in six months is just lying. The problem is, as two experts (Herman and Oster, 2020) point out, that even when the cases decrease considerably it would be difficult to claim unequivocally that it has been due to effective vaccines, because the reduction in cases may be due to the long-term impact of non-vaccine countermeasures like quarantine and social distancing.

How dangerous self-proclaimed knowledge and its dissemination from unqualified sources can be is further proved by two more issues: regarding its 'exact origin', even if the virus may be of animal origin, doubts remain (Cyranoski, 2020) whether bats are its sole source and pangolins are its sole disseminators. Also, there is ambiguity (Cereceda, 2020a) even on the issue whether the virus itself is the 'real killer' or it is the immune system damaging vital organs. The predicament is explained in a straightforward way (Cereceda, 2020b):

> The problems with such a fast and widespread pandemic…is that scientists and doctors only understand the virus and the disease it causes while in a state of flux. Knowledge changes almost daily and it's often disseminated through hundreds of preliminary scientific report that doctors on the ground might not have to scour, busy as they are saving lives.

Much in tune with Hamelink, Jeremy Farrar, Director of the pharmaceutical giant, Wellcome Trust, warns (2020) against any false sense of insecurity relating to the containment of the virus. Appreciating the fact that scientists have been working with incredible speed to deepen understanding of the virus he nevertheless observes that the road to eliminating COVID-19 'still contains many unknowns' concerning the mode of evolution of the virus, of generation of immunity and the longevity of the immunity. Farrar also mentions lack of availability of vaccine to stop people getting sick and of a range of different treatments to help them avoid the need for hospitalisation or to prevent their symptoms from worsening while hospitalised. Noting the invasion of new areas by the virus and the possibility of a second round of infection he notes the enormity of the task of generating knowledge about the exit strategy and the associated interventions to change the fundamentals of infection, transmission and illness.

Even the most publicised role of 'lockdown', inalienably connected with the pandemic times, has been subject to arguments in favour and against. Michael Levitt, a Nobel laureate structural biologist at the Stanford School of Medicine, expressed strong scepticism, based on statistical calculations, about its success. Explaining 'flattening the curve', a phrase widely used to refer to the declining incidents and rate of infection, he points out that it is a result of some degree of prior immunity and large number of asymptomatic cases. Levitt refutes the more prevalent explanation that the flattening is a result of social distancing and lockdowns. He comes up with examples of China, South Korea, Iran and Italy to get home the point. Contrary to the widespread criticism of Sweden, which, as already noted, did not impose lockdown, he praises the Swedish policymakers for getting enough people infected and thus ensuring herd instinct to combat the spread of the pandemic. For him, being less obsessive with lockdown Sweden and Germany became the 'standout winners' in the fight against the virus. By the same logic Levitt criticised Austria, Australia and Israel for losing the plot by pursuing strict lockdown despite having few cases. As for Britain, he finds the country committing a 'huge mistake' in making a shift from the right direction of avoiding lockdown to the wrong direction in being serious about its implementation. Levitt's contentions went straight against the hypothesis of Neil Ferguson, a British epidemiologist, who made very pessimistic forecast about the virus' power of taking lives and strongly advocated the case for lockdown. According to one observer (Carter, 2020), the now discredited Ferguson thesis, with casualty rate being much less than what he had predicted, unravels the limitations of science, including those of epidemiology, a discipline which gets maximum attention and credibility in public sphere. Ferguson's scepticism about the effectiveness of lockdown, however, found some support in the stance of a theoretical epidemiologist at Oxford University, Sunetra Gupta. She points out (Gupta, 2020) that for all practical purposes lockdown can only be imposed for a very limited period and that there is no evident proof that lifting it would inevitably lead to a spurt in infection. In any case, the Ferguson episode proves that even the most experienced scientists are not immune from the perils of wrong and inaccurate predictions. The 'unknown' may induce some to take a swift step to transform it into the 'known' but the outcome runs the risk of being just the opposite of the intention. However, Levitt does not become an uncontested winner when he asserted that the impact of the pandemic was going downwards. In a counterclaim (Leaders, 2020) based on evidence gathered from 84 countries and published in *The Economist* researchers of the Massachusetts Institute of Technology (MIT) noted that the worst was to yet to come. The second wave of the pandemic has proved them right. It has been found by them that for each recorded case of the pandemic 12 go unrecorded and that for every two COVID-19 deaths counted a third is misattributed to other causes. The MIT team also mentioned that without a medical breakthrough the total number of cases would climb to 200 million to 600 million by spring 2021, with the possible deaths reaching a figure between 1.4 million and 3.7 million. A gloomy forecast was also made that during the same time well over 90% of the world's population would still be vulnerable to infection – even more if immunity turns out to be transient.

The dialectics of known and unknown in the specific context of the pandemic seeks to address a generally neglected area of much importance: abundance and overflow of information amidst impoverishment of imperfect and imprecise data. Chapter 5 of the book is exclusively devoted to the emergent phenomenon of infodemic to highlight this development. Here it may be mentioned that governing COVID-19 effectively, with the ultimate goal being the elimination of the virus, is overwhelmingly dependent on the communicative dimensions of governance. Chapters 2 and 3 shall deal with the communicative aspects of the pandemic governance in much detail. Let me briefly mention here that the discovery of effective vaccines or some antidotes is a necessary but not sufficient condition for giving a tough fight to the pandemic. Adequate time has passed to understand that one way of confronting the virus face-to-face is to adopt 'appropriate behaviour'. But it is most certainly a slippery slope. It is so not just because a consensual definition of appropriateness is elusive but also because, as we shall see particularly in Chapter 4, the ruling forces may manipulate 'appropriate behaviour' to enforce conformist behaviour without traces of dissent as part of a more ambitious scheme of regimentation. Communication indeed has a vital role in seeking to effect behavioural change, but the process is not without riders. The aforementioned feature (Leaders, 2020) in *The Economist* explains the predicament in these words:

> Changing behaviour requires clear communication from trusted figures, national and local. But many people do not believe their politicians. In countries, such as, America, Iran, Britain, Russia and Brazil, which have the highest caseloads, presidents and prime ministers minimised the threat, vacillated, issued bad advice or seemed more interested in their own political fortunes than in their country – sometimes all at once.

It also finds that after the initial panic many are becoming disenchanted and resistant to suggestions and advice. Masks are believed to have helped contain the disease, but it is found that in Europe and America there are people refusing to wear one because they see them as emasculating or, worse, a symbol of undemocratic imposition. There is much legitimacy to the claim that though hand washing kills the virus old habits die hard. Congregation of people defying 'social distancing' in parties is known to be dangerous but after a point with the pandemic fatigue setting in one finds the spread of a devil-may-care attitude among the youth. Most important, the feature contends that as the months drag on people just need to earn some money, which leads to defying the restrictive norms.

Such narratives in the context of the pandemic reinforce the point that communication is not just a means to facilitate governing techniques. It plays a key mediating role in defining the nature, extent and efficacy of governance. It is also important to note that communication in this context is a much broader process incorporating media and digital technology within its fold, but it is certainly not limited to them. It inescapably includes people-centric circulation of messages, ideas, opinions, perspectives and beliefs – both from the rulers and from the ruled. In so being, communication is political to the core – in the sense of aiding simultaneous mediation on two counts – 'to' the people and 'from' the people. The pandemic times made us all the more conscious that any complacency about effectiveness of technocratic communication is thoroughly inadequate and would only aggravate the problem. Technocratic approaches thrive on strict stipulations of a series of dos and don'ts for people, often backed up solidly by expertspeak to project the impression of greater legitimacy. In a more specific form they establish a link with risk communication and crisis communication (Chapter 4 will be concerned with these themes). Here suffice is to mention that the limitations of the technocratic approaches to communication are not going unnoticed, as is evident from the following stance (Smith and Judd, 2020:158) seeking to privilege health equity and social justice:

> In health promotion, we need new strategies to communicate important health messages in a concise and meaningful way that makes it easy and accessible for citizens to understand, navigate and take action. We also need to be careful how we convey content through electronic communication channels and consider an appropriate level of frequency of such communication to achieve optimal impact. Without doing so, there is potential to reinforce community ambivalence at one end of the spectrum and create panic at the other.

As will be explained in Chapters 4 and 5, howsoever sophisticated these forms are they are fundamentally meant to give rise to regimented behaviour with lot of biopolitical measures. Therefore, they go a long way to prove, often contrary to their objectives, that politics is inscribed in communication itself and any attempt to prove otherwise is misleading.

No one denies the long-standing role of the state in the context of epidemics and pandemics. McMillen (p. 5) for one affirms a clear connection between epidemics/ pandemics and the growth of the modern state, and traces it back to the fifteenth century when in response to the plague the Italian city states formed state-sponsored boards of health. (The role of Leonardo da Vinci has already been mentioned in the Introduction). McMillen also writes that the cholera pandemics of the nineteenth century led to nationwide efforts at quarantine – efforts that could only be carried off by a central state. He also adds that measures, such as, compulsory vaccination also demonstrated this connection. But the issue is that the state cannot do it effectively without some forms of communication – be it then and be it now.

Governance beyond doubt is a complex affair[2] and in the next chapter its elemental and contextual aspects will be critically taken up. Governance confronts a bewildering variety of situations and needs careful handling of the same. There is no linear way of negotiation and the pandemic situation makes it even more evident. In an interesting account Nick Chater (2020) comes up with a typology of interpretations of the challenges of the pandemic, faced by governments. They are variously termed as 'storm in a tea-cup', 'house on fire' and 'holding back the tide'. The first kind is described as the mind's natural default: most alarms are false alarms; most panics are overblown. This does not obviously preclude the current pandemic. The examples pertinent to this genre are China's attempt to suppress information, the initial underestimation of the pandemic by US and Britain, and also the contentions of some leading scholars and researchers mentioned earlier in the discussion. This type of interpretation conveys the point that the problem is not only manageable but also resolvable, and that there is no need to be panic stricken about the pandemic. The 'house on fire' kind, led by the idea that the virus is to be tackled with utmost urgency and with top priority, includes the instances of unprecedented degree of lockdowns in China, South Korea, some European countries and India. Chater explains that the economic and social impacts of the lockdown will be vast but have to be endured, rather like collateral water damage, however severe, caused by the firefighter's hose. This also implies that taking the strongest action as the 'right time to start fighting a fire is: immediately!' The third kind, of 'holding back the tide', sees beating down the virus as workable only as a temporary stop-gap. It is based on the assumption that there can be only temporary defence against the rising tide, but inundation is unavoidable. In precise terms, eradication being impossible the way forward should be to avoid aggressive countermeasures and the adoption of a staged approach to minimise the impact and wait for herd immunity to occur in course of time. Chater mentions the danger of sticking to one particular form of interpretation, with the implicit logic that changing nature of knowledge warranted by changing circumstances proves the futility of rigid adherence to any one kind. Apart from the uncertainties in the epidemiological and clinical issues relating to the pandemic, issues of framing and containment concerning risk, about which one expects to have wider agreement, there is a prevailing lack of consensus. A probing review paper (Carney and Bennett, 2014) curating a range of literature from different disciplines confirms this point. The paper mentions (p. 136) that there is as yet little agreement on how risk should be framed – opinions being divided on whether it is a scientific, social or political question. Opinions are also at odds on what kind of governance response is warranted – whether it should prioritise quarantine or should it be public education and public awareness. There is also little consensus on how the pandemic management is perceived or accepted by a culturally diverse public. The review paper also mentions (p. 138) in clear terms that sociological, cultural and political perspectives on the pandemic reveal some of the shortcomings of a 'purely' governance and scientific approach. In another significant observation, keeping the WHO pandemic protocols in the forefront, the paper points out that from a purely legal or governance perspective, the WHO model is a radical departure from the Westphalian theory of harnessing autonomous sovereign states into collaboration through treaties. The root of this transformation is traced to the 'globalised', 'networked', 'nodal' order of sharing of information, thereby bringing national pandemic governance systems into more distributed, complex and polycentric assemblages and arrangements. It is not that the WHO model is being accepted in a friction-free manner, as has been evident in President Trump's histrionics against the UN agency and withdrawal of funding. But the point is that the pandemic governance is exposing several twists and turns vis-à-vis the 'new normal', which are too evident to ignore.

All these issues and developments may be related to the unfolding of the (neoliberal) governance thesis as constructed and promoted in the global era since the early 1990s – a point to be discussed in the next chapter. In this design the prime role of the market and high legitimacy accorded to profit motive are to be underlined. Yet, the government/state-market relations are not as smooth as it is generally assumed. On the contrary in certain cases the relations assume myriad forms. An example from India reveals how complex it is. On 2 July, 2020, the Director General of the Indian Council for Medical Research (ICMR) wrote to twelve select trial sites asking them to begin clinical trials of COVAXIN, a COVID-19 vaccine developed by Hyderabad-based Bharat Biotech. The overzealous drive is to be attributed to the lack of patience to wait for the outcome of human clinical trials of the vaccine by the Drugs Controller General of India. (A newspaper cartoon showed a scientist on the top of a mountain standing on one leg in a yogi position and praying to the Almighty to help him to meet the deadline!). The letter pressed for quick 'public health use' by 15 August – the Indian Independence Day. It is also the day when by way of a convention the Indian Prime Minister addresses the nation from the Red Fort, which includes listing the achievements of the central government. In the face of virulent criticism in political and media circles, of the way the target date has been set for the researchers, couple of days later the ICMR issued a statement that the date was fixed as a message to get rid of red-tapism without bypassing any necessary steps in the process of discovery of the antiviral. What it reveals is that the concern for civilian biodefence is often a convenient tool for political publicity and rhetoric, and as will be discussed in Chapter 4, it is an effective tool of biopolitics. The instance may also be linked to the compulsive acceleration inscribed in 'good governance' and its credo of efficiency in the neoliberal times, a theme which I have extensively discussed elsewhere (Sinha, 2021:30–58). Some researchers of pandemic politics are not, however, surprised with this kind of development. In a study of the pharmaceutical politics during pandemic times Stefan Elbe (2018:2) finds particularly in the governments of this century a political aspiration of having a line-up of 'medical countermeasures'. These measures are readily available for public distribution to prevent an outbreak, and more importantly for our discussion here, when the outbreak is caused by a new disease and the governments insist on having the capability to rapidly develop *new* medical countermeasures in response. Elbe notes that governments face serious and protracted obstacles in such effort, mainly sourced from a clash of two logics: a political/security logic whereby they wish to secure people against emerging biological dangers, and a commercial market logic that prefers a wait and watch policy which does not naturally prioritise the costly development of such products without having a more clearly defined market. It is certainly not an easy situation for governments because of the dominance of commercial logic in the global pharmaceutical industry. Elbe also finds (p. 230) no immediate solution to the problem because governments are finding it hard to find 'critical distance', some kind of engagement with the pharmaceutical companies without being too close to them – an approach which would find credibility in public perception. With the growing clout of the market forces and their relentless pursuit of profit any health crisis becomes a great impetus for profit generation. (A cartoon in India conveys the reality graphically when it depicts corporate hospitals drawing juice from the coronavirus, with pharmaceutical companies waiting eagerly with a big bucket).

Flexi-modern phenomenon

Let me now extrapolate some key attributes of the classic theorisation of 'late' modernity (3) and try to relate them to the pandemic times. 'Late' has close connect with prefixes like 'high', 'reflexive', 'second' when it comes to the critical theories of modernity. Keeping crisis, risk, anxiety and panic in the background of late modernity I prefer to describe the coronavirus pandemic as a flexi-modern development. The pandemic as a flexi-modern phenomenon generates a semi-fluid state of the contemporary world as it is. My argument is that it is anchored in the parameters of modernity but not exactly in a rigid and monochromatic way. The following discussion would make it clear that even if the formulation depends on the conceptual frameworks of late modernity the analytical frame makes a light departure from it. It is too well known that the later phase of modernity has been impressively theorised by Bauman (2000), Beck (1992) and Giddens (1990) among others. However, one may not venture to go the extent of calling it a totally fluid/liquid scenario. The pandemic has perhaps created the greatest disruption ever to the modern institutions and cultures, but it has not yet acquired enough force to usher in a totally fluid situation to warrant a great leap forward to the next stage of social existence. It is very turbulent times for the 'modern' civilisation but rather than dissolving everything around us the times beckon us to rethink and reframe some of our obsessive thoughts and actions and reset ourselves. One possible way is to discard complacency about our acquired knowledge and embark on the twin processes of rethinking and reframing by according importance to uncertainty.

Though constitutively it may not be so, modernity is generally promoted as a crust made of 'rational', 'objective', 'scientific', 'secular' and 'specialised' order of institutions and 'appropriate' cultural configurations. Yet there is a difference between what is the original, ideal and mandated form of modernity, the master plan as constructed by the Enlightenment philosophy, and what it becomes in course of its journey in existential world by facing trials, tribulations, encounters, resistances, aberrations and the consequent adaptations to the challenging situations. The details of such trajectory of modernity are beyond the immediate scope of this book but it may be noted that the beauty of modernity is that while it faces numerous challenges on its way it survives in one way or the other. On the specific issue of 'flexibility' there is no claim on my part that what is being flagged here is an earth shatteringly new hypothesis. Ample hints have been provided about it in the analyses of modernity in terms of 'ambivalence' and 'counter-modernisation' (Bauman, 1991, 1997). Here, I am only trying to explore the issue in the specific context of COVID-19. Bauman, widely considered to be the chief priest of the liquid modernity thesis, however, mentions (2000:3) that his idea has its roots much before him – among other instances in the well-quoted phrase 'melting the solids' in *The Communist Manifesto*. But Bauman is to be given credit for famously theorising the 'liquefaction' factor in modernity, drawing attention to its fluidity and lightness and even pointing out that it had been incorporated in modernity from the very beginning. He offers (Bauman, 2000:2) a very significant statement highlighting the nature of fluids: 'Fluids travel easily. They 'flow', 'spill', 'run out', 'splash', 'pour over', 'leak', 'flood', 'spray', 'drip', 'seep', 'ooze'; unlike solids, they are not easily stopped – they pass around some obstacles, dissolve some others and bore or soak their way through others still.' The series of acts mentioned in the statement reveals the difference between fluids and solids. As the background of his analysis of emancipation, individuality, time/space, work and community the following excerpt from Bauman (2000:7) succinctly describes the process of reconfiguration:

> These days patterns and configurations are no longer 'given', let alone 'self-evident'; there are just too many of them, clashing with one another and contradicting one another's commandments, so that each one has been stripped of a good deal of compelling, coercively constraining powers. And they have changed their nature and have been accordingly reclassified: as items in the inventory of individual tasks. Rather than preceding life-politics and framing its future course, they are to follow it (follow from it), to be shaped and reshaped by its twists and turns. The liquidizing powers have moved from the 'system' to 'society', from politics' to 'life-policies' – or have descended from the 'macro' to the 'micro' level of social cohabitation.

In the present context, taking us further from where Bauman had left Young (2007:1–16) discusses 'the vertigo of modernity' and relates the fluidity norms to a host of factors such as mass migration and tourism, labour, breakdown of community, instability of family, rise of virtual realities, proliferation and speed of media. These factors to him are the means of cultural globalisation, impact of mass consumerism, and the idealisation of individualism, choice, and spontaneity. Young also marks the presence of ontological insecurity – in the precariousness of being – in such potential for flexibility and reinvention. He writes that at no stage in history has there been such a premium on identity, on constructing a narrative of development and discovery, yet where the materials to construct it are so transient and insubstantial. At the same time he finds that fluidity can create the possibilities of seeing through the present institutional set up, of discarding the old traditions, of respect for authority justifying the status quo, of wealth and social division. Side by side, he also refers to the global implosion of media imagery and actual realities, which produces at the most a sense of disorientation and points to the possibility that things could be different, and that rational discourse need not lead to the same conclusions as in one's own culture. He adds that it de-reifies and de-familiarises – making the familiar no longer obvious and taken for granted. Though Young repeatedly refers to the American lower and middle classes to get through his point he acknowledges that his contentions might have broader social relevance. I would complement Young's contentions by stating that his formulations of the 'vertigo' in the era of COVID-19 has broader relevance even beyond the shores of America and it can also be situated, while incorporating it, beyond his prime area of concern – politics of identity. The experience of insecurities in particular, born out of uncertainties, has been linked by him to the vertigo of the 'ne'er-do-wells' outside of the 'charmed sphere of the contented minority'. In Young's view, vertigo as the 'malaise of late modernity' harbours a constellation of trends and symptoms: a sense of insecurity of insubstantiality, and of uncertainty, a whiff of chaos and a fear of falling. The signs of giddiness, of unsteadiness, are everywhere, some serious, many minor; yet once acknowledged, a series of separate seemingly disparate facts begin to fall into place. The obsession with rules, an insistence on clear uncompromising lines of demarcation between correct and incorrect behaviour, a narrowing of borders, the decreased tolerance of deviance, a disproportionate response to rule-breaking, an easy resort to punitiveness and a point at which simple punishment begins to verge on the vindictive (p. 12). Above all, his contentions indicate that binary vision is under severe strain with hyper-pluralism and hybridity. Blurred, shifting and detached boundaries are becoming the 'new normal', to use a popular lexicon dominating our life in the pandemic times. (As it is said now, not acknowledging the 'new normal' is abnormal!) The predicament not only concerns philosophy, humanities and social sciences but also science itself. Justifying why COVID-19 as 'post-normal' pandemic requires a new approach in science a number of concerned scholars continue to raise a set of pertinent questions. A quote from one such scholar (Waltner-Toews et al., 2020) may further explain their position:

> The new, still-emerging social contract calls on us to pause in our vocal desperation to make square peg of normal science fit the round hole for which it was never intended, and to re-shape our activities to fit the new reality. But what if we experience, this time, more so than previously, that we are not in control? Are we condemned to do "more of the same" forever until we're

forced to do something else by the events (because of a collapse)? It is time to raise valid questions, rather than seeking solutions in haste.

My conceptual stance on 'flexi-modernity' may require some explanations of my stance on postmodernism. Though deeply appreciative the epistemic alert raised by postmodernism there is reason to agree with the comment (Cahoone 1996:2) that it deserves careful, sober scrutiny, devoid of trendy enthusiasm, indignant condemnation, or reactionary fear. It is especially so because the postmodern thoughts have varied origins and a bewildering range of intellectual streams (for a summary, Best and Kellner, 1991). Also, one may recollect a highly provocative comment by Lyotard (1984:79) that postmodernism is 'undoubtedly part of the modern'. While many hitherto 'sacrosanct' truths are coming under scrutiny and the inherent power relations are being shaken the progressivist core of modernity is not yet weak enough to be discarded log, stock and barrel. The structures, institutions and frameworks of modernity do have 'fragments' but they are yet to be superseded by counter-forces. In such new configurations, which can be described as a shift from downright hostility to strategic collaboration, the state and market are lending new dynamics 'late' phase to modernity and contributing to its flexibility impulse. A number of events and issues of such collaboration will come up in the ensuing discussion in the book.

Among its various lessons the COVID-19 pandemic has also made us aware of the need to adopt caution in describing in a 'postmodern vein' that all scientific truths as nothing more than social constructions. This is not to deny that science has a fair share of relativity and subjectivity. The above discussion has provided evidence of scientists themselves being increasingly open to the relative and subjective nature of their propositions. But swift act of equating scientific contentions with myths calls for caution. It will surely lead to a science versus social science face-off in some ways, a development least desirable in such crisis times when some transdisciplinary or cross-disciplinary epistemic engagements with inter-stream tolerance are of immense importance with regard to various issues of common concern and public welfare. Even while accepting that 'facts' are being constructed especially in the era of systematic mis/disinformation, and that there is a strong need to ensure contestabil of facts in the light of what the postmodernists identify as contextual, contingent subject positions and strategic locations it may not be all that easy to unhesitatingly confirm that 'there is no such thing as fact'. Numerous counterfactual images, signals and spectacles do engulf the world around us and they intensify their operations during the pandemic but they do not necessarily negate the facts; they at best overshadow them. The exploration of the known-unknown dialectics in such tumultuous times can be best addressed with a good dose flexible approaches on the part of all. Here in lies the rationale of flexi-modern approach.

Concluding remarks

The discussion so far affirms that if there is any colour of the COVID-19 pandemic it is 'grey'. In spite of repeated claims of 'growing clarity' about the nature of the coronavirus/pandemic and of 'transparency' in its governance there are much too unknown elements contributing to the incomplete knowledge. There is no one-size-fits-all solution understanding of the pandemic and if such a solution is sought it is bound to have an adverse impact on the exploration of knowledge about the phenomenon. In scientific research (including epidemiological profiling), social scientific inquiry, policy design, and in the decision-making and service delivery process hasty claims of 'crystal clear' views may produce negative consequences. This remains true despite the pandemic being at the centre stage of loads of statistics, metrics, models, techniques and guidelines, which are being relentlessly created and promoted.

It is true that no one wishes to celebrate the occurrence of a grave tragedy. But the problem as shown by the coronavirus pandemic is that despite a multitude of stakeholders participating and performing simultaneously to achieve the common goal of containing and eradicating the scourge too many contradictions, ambiguities and vagueness remain in both thinking and action. Even when the pandemic goes away, if it does at all, no one would be able to claim that everything was known about it. 'Complete knowledge' of the virus and the pandemic is like, to borrow from Confucius, searching for a non-existent black cat in a dark room. 'We know' is the most ideal assertion but 'we just don't know enough' is the more practical one. The pandemic has perhaps taught us a hard lesson which does not necessarily generate a comfortable feeling: that we have to live with its unknown elements and the fragility of our ideas for an indeterminate period of time.

Notes

1 The newest entry in this league is 'green swan' which in the specific context of climate change refers to unexpected environmental catastrophe in the form of global warming and/or pollution with the distinct possibility of endangering lives and livelihoods. In the ensuing discussion I shall refer to the black swan metaphor in some detail in taking up the known-unknown dialectics.

2 Explicating governance in functionalist terms and specifying its requirements of success Guy Peters (2012:22) refers to a set of activities. The way he puts them provides a number of hints about the complexity and strategic flexibility about it. The four activities are: a) Goal Selection: Governing is steering and steering requires some knowledge about the destination toward which one is steering – a task that may need a wide range of social actors. Goals being very complex affair – multi-layered, broad as well as operational, effective governance requires the integration of goals across all levels of the systems; b) Goal Reconciliation and Coordination: The multiple actors within government all have their own goals, and effective governance therefore requires establishing some priorities and coordinating the actions taken according to those priorities; c) Implementation: The decisions made in the first two stages of the process above must then be put into effect, requiring some form of implementation. Peters reiterate that this stage of the process is more likely to can be performed by state actors but it may also involve social actors; and finally, d) Feedback and Accountability: Individuals and institutions involved in governance need to learn from their actions. This is important both for improving the quality of the decisions being made and also for democratic accountability. Therefore, some well-developed method of feedback must be built into the governance arrangements.

2

'GOVERNANCING' CONTAGION

Lockdown or meltdown?

Introduction

Much like what is said of justice, governance must not only be done but it must also appear to be done. But COVID-19 has proved that it is not necessarily the case. It is an open secret that the actually existing governance, if I may put it that way, has been put under severest strain by the pandemic due to a constellation of events which no one could predict. Ever since the outbreak too many governments have failed their own people, that too with dire and long-lasting consequences. Even the countries which are traditionally regarded as the 'best governed', those which usually take immense pride in proclaiming themselves as so and many of which preach their 'less efficient' counterparts a long lesson in good governance, now face the ignominy of under-performance, if not non-performance. Ironical it may sound, when it comes to managing the pandemic a number of hitherto 'achiever' states have come to acquire many of the traits of the habitually branded 'failed' states. COVID-19 exposes the weaknesses of (good) governance in almost all the countries of the world. The grim pandemic scenario reminded one of the supposed conversation between two top civil servants in the classic British sitcom, *Yes, Minister*, in which four successive acts are delineated for the unprepared prime minister to follow: Stage 1: We say nothing is going to happen; Stage 2: We say something may be about to happen, but we should do nothing about it; Stage 3: We say that maybe we should do something about it, but there's nothing we can do; Stage 4: we say maybe there was something we could have done, but it's too late now. On 12 March 2020, The Independent, a British online daily, resonated the satirical view of some Twitter users by linking these stages to the Prime Minister Boris Johnson's reaction to the pandemic. But it might be unfair to single him out as he seems to have a number of counterparts adopting the similar approach in different parts of the world. Pandemic governance seems to have involved the art of doing little.

DOI: 10.4324/9781003247388-3

In this context, India, by becoming the epicentre of the second wave of the coronavirus, demands special mention. While the country earned the dubious first rank in terms of the number of infected people and in the number of deaths the central and state governments displayed an alarming blend of indifference and confusion in tackling the second strain of the virus. A false sense of security led to a highly premature official declaration of the 'victory over the virus', which turned out to be more of a catchphrase. Complacent attitude about the relative success in meeting the first wave combined with populism and demagoguery to result in complete unpreparedness. Despite having gained some respite between the first and the second waves of the pandemic no care was taken to formulate a national COVID policy in India. With the outbreak of the more deadly second strain the mutual blame game between the central government and several state governments reached its peak, only to succeed in making ordinary people the worst victims of the crisis. The situation became unmanageably grave with long-time reluctance to increase budgetary investment in basic healthcare. In times of the crisis it resulted in lack of hospital beds, life-saving medicines and oxygen supply. Deaths and sufferings all around, accompanied by lack of transparent vaccination policy, led to a severe trust deficit among people, with adverse impact on legitimacy and effectiveness of governance.

Before moving further into the discussion it may be clarified that the term 'governance' in this book connotes a specific link with the neoliberal paradigm. Governance has been one of the most recurring themes in social science literature since the 1990s. Its origin, parameters and forms are being theorised with great enthusiasm over the last three decades.[1] In a compact form it implies 'steering' or 'managing' rather than administering in the conventional mode, with much dominant role of the market and the irreversibly lesser, if not downright minimal, role ('rollback'/'downsizing') of the state divested of its long monopoly over expertise and resources. Here I shall be more concerned with the state and fate of 'governance', though not in the broad dictionary-specific meaning of action or manner of governing. As already hinted, it is a concept, and not just a term, which is endowed with a specific context of emergence at a particular juncture of time in accordance with certain pathos delineated by transnational institutions like the World Bank and the UNDP (United Nations Development Programme) as the ideological and empirical progenitors. 'Governance' here will also be intimately linked to the radical concept of 'good governance', a dominant but controversial term in the contemporary discourses of governing and development. 'Governance' will also be linked to both 'governing' and 'government', and with the much dicey issue of governability – indicating the capacity of the system and actors involved in the act of governing – in the background. 'Governing' will be used in a more generic sense to describe what governments do or are supposed to do – as distinct from 'governancing' which is governance-specific. Another concept, 'governmentality', which has distinctive power-knowledge equations and a tie-up with 'governance' in terms of monitoring and surveillance, will be part of the discussion in the next chapter.

The purpose of this chapter is to argue that notwithstanding the abstract conceptual-theoretical endeavours to revisit and somewhat reframe the ideational elements of governance in the face of periodic challenges and mounting critiques the empirically driven actually existing form of governance – governance-as-it-is/governance-in-practice – remains too strategic, codified, technocratic and decontextualised and prone to underperformance. The crisis situation created by the COVID-19 pandemic has made it all the more visible. I shall flag the point that 'governance' is a light entity with lot of ideational frills but with little effectiveness in terms of the welfare of people, but I would not venture to announce its death-knell. The reason will be revealed subsequently.

There is little scope for disagreement if it is argued that the coronavirus-led pandemic has provided a highly challenging scenario when it comes to the interplay of the concepts mentioned earlier. It is not that in the pre-pandemic years the interplay was non-existent. But there is no doubt that in the twentieth year of the current millennium it has produced a bewildering array of diversity, complexity and dynamics. COVID-19 has affected more than 180 countries and it is only obvious that each country has a governing system of its own. But when it comes to the entity of governments in the structural sense there are various layers at the national, regional and local levels. Besides there are other vectors like the largely amorphous concept of 'global governance' and a more niche variety like corporate governance. The question that demands exploration is how does the pandemic confront governance and how does 'governance' respond. Long ago, Robert Dahl (1961) with his limited focus on an American city administration had raised a brief but a most significant question – 'who governs?', connecting it to the tricky issues of powerplay and democracy. Confronted with a much larger canvas and much broader horizons in the pandemic situation there is every reason at this moment to take up the question with vigour, supplementing it with the exploration of the mode and mechanisms of governing.

(Good) Governance: tested negative

The numerous hotspots marked by the free play of COVID-19 are putting governments throughout the world in a spot. Judging from the developments it may be presumed that there is no definite timeline within which the 'post pandemic era' in the true sense of the term would emerge. The threat of coronavirus with no specific expiry date, and its survival even in a low transmission mode, raise many issues about the nature of governing. At the foundational level it questions the efficacy of the nation-states, especially of their public policies and particularly with policies and strategies regarding public health and social security. On a broader scale it has also brought under scanner a host of issues concerning rights, freedoms, privacy, security and so forth. Governments are in near-total disarray and ordinary people are in dismay as to how to negotiate with the pandemic situation. The problem is that there is no clarity about the functioning of the nation-states through national, international and global channels. The depth and spread of the pandemic have adversely affected whatever clarity about their trajectory was claimed in scholarly discourses and in their everyday practice. If one still subscribes to the Westphalian genre of nation-states and organised political community one is bound to be not only confused but also clueless with the virus threatening this long-established order from the bottom. If on the other hand one is a strict proponent of the Washington consensus, the so-called seed of the neoliberal paradigm advocating 'post-welfare' economic, financial and fiscal discipline with 'minimum government, maximum governance', the situation is not radically different either.

The focus on (good) governance here is to be attributed to the fact that having passed more than three decades since its emergence and advocacy of the neoliberal policies, and having the advantage of the absence of any credible alternatives, its score card has been highly disappointing. In fact, it tested negative when it comes to its capability of handling the disruptions caused by the outbreak. Analysts like Mark Bevir (2010:1) recognises the fact that 'governance' is a vague and contested concept and finds it unfortunate that its ubiquity does not make its meaning any clearer and that a lack of clarity about its meaning might engender scepticism about its importance. He explains that lack of clarity about what governance is lends piquancy to the following questions: How does the concept differ from that of government? Why has the concept become ubiquitous? What is its relationship to democracy? How do policy actors respond to its challenges? Scanning the literature on governance Bevir also finds (p. 3) an exhibition of three cardinal ideas: i) that the state is fragmented, consisting of self-interested actors or complex networks; ii) that social science explains policy outcomes by appealing to formal ahistorical models, correlations, mechanisms, or processes; and iii) that representative institutions are at most a small part of a larger policy process in which a range of actors, many of whom are unelected and unaccountable, negotiate, formulate and implement policies in accord with their particular interests and norms. The discussion here will seek to address these questions by situating them in the pandemic scenario, but more in a spirit of exploration than in a solution-centric vein.

The pandemic has shown that all is not at all well with its supposed pillars of 'good governance' – accountability, transparency, responsiveness and the most flaunted one, efficiency. The problem is compounded by the fact that those who look for a viable alternative are still in the dark. Without indulging in a debate whether ideologies are smokescreens to confuse and exploit people it can be argued that neither overarching ideologies nor tailor-made, ready-to-serve strategies are making any sense or having any use when it comes to the crucial questions of combating the virus and saving people from death, depression and enormous insecurity of economic and social kinds. Globalisation was for a long time in aggressive peak promising a better world order, but the pandemic has made sure that its emancipatory and transformatory promises sound hollow. But even when some scholars make the right move they might be going the wrong way. Let me take one example. One tends to agree with Dani Rodrik (2020) that hyper-globalisation has become 'defensive'. But it is difficult to agree with his easy diagnosis – that the nation-states are trying to reclaim policy space and that neoliberalism is witnessing a 'slow death'. Incidentally, he also underplays the power of the pandemic when he argues that no one should expect it to alter, much less reverse, the tendencies that were evident before the crisis.

The main point is that the knowledge constructed and publicised globally vis-à-vis the thesis-cum-diktat of governance has been found to be largely ineffective, if not fruitless, to counter the pandemic. The viral aggression shows that there was little preparation to tackle it because none had any clue about its coming. Even when one does not absolve China for being in some way responsible for putting the world in such grave situation the fact remains that just by blaming the country with a different political system and an 'adverse' political ideology may serve the purpose of political battle. But it does not fully explain why despite the duration of (good) governance for a fairly long time we are witnessing its failure on multiple fronts across the world. In this context there is much food for thought in Merlee Grindle periodic revisits of the (good) governance agenda. In the early years of this century she had flagged (2004:525–526) a crucial point that 'not surprisingly advocating good governance raises a host of questions about what needs to be done, when it needs to be done, and how it needs to be done'. Alongside, she introduced the concept of 'good enough governance', which is supposed to provide a platform for questioning the long menu of institutional changes and capacity-building initiatives currently deemed important or essential for development. Six years later, Grindle (2010) would further qualify the point by asserting that 'governance' seems to be an inflated idea. Describing the concept as 'seductive' and the 'new kid in development discourse' she noted that it needs to be reformatted on the basis of a reasonable understanding of what 'good governance' can deliver and what it cannot. Calling peers to be careful and advocating scepticism as an intellectual tool to check inflation of such concepts Grindle identified (2010:15) three sources of the problem of inflation of the concept of governance: i) Development – whether economic or political–is a long-term and complex process; research is far from understanding the timing and the complexity of 'getting developed'; ii) Explorations of historical experience can do much to illuminate issues of timing and complexity; and iii) When concepts like governance take on strong normative content, such as good governance, their importance and impact attract researchers, practitioners and advocates, who in turn may add to the process of conceptual inflation.

Interestingly, the COVID-19 pandemic has proved Grindle right beyond what she was analytically contemplating. Her analysis made a distinction between the developed and developing states – with the argument that the latter were more at the receiving end of not-so-good governance. The pandemic in unleashing its impact has made the distinction blurred. By 2011 she revisited the concept of good governance and found it was high time to introduce the concept of 'good enough governance'. She continued from her earlier contention about the predicaments and challenges of (good) governance and identified a foundational problem in the definitional stage itself when she states (2011:S201, italics in the original text) the following:

> In moving from the definition of governance to that of *good* governance, normative views of what 'ought to be' become even more prominent. Yet definitions vary in the degree to which they imply particular policies or policy outcomes – stable macroeconomic policy, reduction of poverty, openness to trade, decentralisation, or efficient revenue collection, for example – or particular institutional forms and processes – democracy, widespread participation in development decision-making, or strong legislatures, for example. Moreover, given such broad definitions, it is often not clear how governance can be distinguished from development itself.

She also observed that beyond the definitional concerns about governance and good governance there lies a contentious debate about issues like measurement, indicators and inference. Within six years Grindle (2017) seemed to have lost any hope of reforming possibilities of the good governance agenda when she came out with a brief article wryly titled 'Good Governance, RIP: A Critique and an Alternative'. It clearly showed that insofar as her scheme is concerned the days of 'good governance' are over. The article contained important truths about the 'good governance', which are helpful in understanding to a significant extent why governance in the pandemic situation lands itself up in such confusing state of affairs. At the very outset of the discussion she clearly mentioned that research and practice over the past two decades suggested that conceptually good governance 'more often obscures than enlightens'. It grew to become an 'impossibly inflated idea' and being too much embedded in a specific idea of development, implying the neoliberal variety, it has itself become uncertain to the extent of ultimately being a source of 'muddy thinking' about the role of government in the development process. The major problem she found was that being so inflated and fused with popularity it went on to mask a more critical issue in governance – how to change it for the better. She also found little need to consult the idea of good governance in order to increase understanding of how institutions of governance emerge, evolve and sometimes improve. Grindle identified, three years before COVID-19 struck the blow, that notwithstanding the promotion and inflation of good governance in development thinking certain key conditions are yet to be met. The conditions she identified includes equity, participation, inclusiveness, democracy, widespread service delivery, sound regulation, decentralisation, respect for civil and human rights, gender and racial equality, good investment climate, citizen security and job creation. The pandemic has produced enough evidence to argue that all these are being abandoned in the era of good governance. The hold-all concept of good governance, it may be added, stifles the motivation to explore the 'unknown' because of the excessive confidence in the 'known'. It creates a bubble of impregnability around the thesis of good governance with the help of, as will be explained below, disciplinary knowledge and its embedded modes of inquiry. Having an ambitious plan to develop into an all-embracing concept good governance removes all avenues of critical deliberations and debates. Grindle alluded (2017:19) to this while noting that the inflated concept encouraged 'one best way' thinking about what needs to be done, with technical fixes, best practices and adoption of solutions from other contexts, thus helping the lead countries to fall, intentionally or unintentionally, into traps of isomorphic mimicry, in which formal solutions to governance problems are introduced with little regard to their situational fit or impact. This is precisely where the deficiency of the hold-all approach is exposed.

The critical explorations of the polity continue to take sustenance from the pandemic. Describing the coronavirus as 'ideology-agnostic contagion' a commentator (Aiyar, 2020) raises a relevant point that the nature of the pandemic has proved beyond doubt that the political system – democratic or coercive authoritarian – plays a secondary role in determining the success rate of a nation's response. The key, she finds, not in the form of government but in its efficiency, nimbleness, openness to learning and in the ability to adapt best practices to local circumstances. About the high success rate in containing the pandemic she refers to the South-East Asian countries like Singapore, South Korea, Taiwan and Hong Kong to explain that while these countries are either far from or not exactly at par with the open societies of the west what they have seriously pursued is the lesson they learnt from the SARS coronavirus crisis of 2002–2003. These countries have been widely commended for effective use of diagnostic and digital technologies to deal with the pandemic. The basic point here is that if the pandemic has exposed the western developed states as thoroughly as many of the non-western developing countries, and if the two 'parallel lines' have met, it is because of the common feature – unwillingness to learn from own experience and from that of others. On this issue one finds a point of view (Khoo, 2020:7–16) which refers to the hierarchical order in the global arena to directly indict the Global North for its indifference to learn lessons from the pandemic experience of the Global South. But this may just be a symptom of a deeper disease that afflicts the Washington Consensus and its 'Golden Straitjacket' form, to borrow a widely quoted term of Milton Friedman (2000:101–111), one of the chief architects of the Washington Consensus. The Golden Straitjacket, a set of economic and financial rules weaved among other things by liberalisation, privatisation and deregulation, is in his description the 'defining political–economic garment' of the globalisation era. Friedman notes that while the Cold War era had more than one jackets like the Mao suit, the Nehru jacket, the Russian fur, this era has only one – 'the only model on the rack'. He then predicted in a now-or-never tenor that if one's country has not been fitted for one, it will be soon. At the same time, according to him, it is 'one-size-fits-all' kind and it is neither pretty nor gentle nor comfortable. Its political economic manoeuvring, one can clearly see from his description, is close ended. He adds that in keeping a society under pressure to constantly streamline its economic institutions and upgrade its performance it reduces political choices down to the level of choice between Pepsi or Coke – permitting 'slight nuances of taste, slight nuances of policy, slight alterations in design to account for local traditions, some loosening here or there, but never any major deviation from the core golden rules'. The 'minor tailoring changes' leave no scope for intense political debates over policies followed. Here Friedman reminds one of Daniel Bells' thesis (Bell, 1960) of the 'end of ideology and the exhaustion of political ideas', which though having its temporal focus on 1950s, was also illustrative of the shrinking space for political debates except for some showcasing absolutely secondary issues. Both scholars, economist Friedman and sociologist Bell, thrive on rhetoric and euphemisms but are straightforward enough to put the message through that the reigning ideology of their respective times are basically a façade of general interest and universal values, but in actuality they are nothing but masks of self-interest. The only difference between the two being Bell's more radical contention of total exhaustion of ideology. To refer to Friedman's discussion of the Golden Straitjacket, he was quite confident that 'the tighter it is worn the more gold it will produce'. Friedman's approach has been critiqued widely and deep scepticism about its success has been expressed but there is no doubt that it has come under severest strain with astonishing directness in the pandemic days. The gold production, whatever it means, was halted and Friedman's supremely confident claims suddenly began to sound like tall claims.

This again brings us to the realm of the known-unknown dialectics. Analysts like Levy-Faur (2012:7) while delineating the theoretical trajectory of governance has insisted on it being a 'signifier of change' by virtue of its supposed ability to carry images and meanings of change in an era of change, shifts and even transformation and paradigm change. But such perspective has a major limitation because the methodology of acquiring and negotiating knowledge in governancing remains a blind spot in it. The greatest impact that shrinking space for political debates regarding governance-induced public policies falls on the 'unknown unknowns'. It is because they are never taken into account by the governance agenda. Or, even if they ever come into cognition they are simply ignored. The problem does not end there. Even when the 'unknown unknowns' make appearance to a certain degree to become inevitably known the players in governance remain totally unprepared because they had remained unrehearsed. Taking a jibe at critics who had ridiculed Rumsfeld and dismissed his known/unknown thesis one observer (Alles, 2009:88) looks for a better sense with these words:

> ...whether one calls it an unknown unknown, ambiguity, fat tails or black swans, it is essential that those of us in the governance arena start to develop practices that makes us contemplate the unthinkable and prepare to deal with events that are not just the worst-case scenario, but worse than what we can even imagine. Only then will we have the assurance that we have done everything possible to cope with everything that is possible.

My own contention is that such dawning of better sense is ideal but not something to be realised easily if one considers the essential parameters and policy imperatives of the (good) governance agenda.

The (good) governance agenda comes with many promises, but it remains totally indifferent to the multi-layered dialectics of the known-unknown, thereby side-tracking the unavoidable overlapping of knowledge and ignorance. As a result, it undermines the importance of risks. Chapter 5 will take up the risk communication issue in greater detail but a preliminary discussion can be fruitful at this stage. Taking the cue from the discussion in Chapter 1 let me in this context refer to the four quadrants – knowledge, risks, untapped knowledge and uncertainty. Developed by Cleden (2009:12–15) in the specific context of strategisation of project management it has far broader relevance. First, knowledge is known knowns. It is composed of predictable future states, data and independently verifiable evidence. Second, there are risks – the known unknowns. It is composed of possible states identified, ambiguous outcomes, quantifiable variables and known contingency actions. Third, there is the untapped knowledge – the unknown knowns. It comprises researchable facts, unshared skills and information and untapped resources. Fourth, there is uncertainty – the unknown unknowns. In this case the components are hidden knowledge, unknown relationships evidence between key variables, unpredictable events and the sudden phenomenon described as 'bolts from the blue'. Cleden calls it the Four Quadrants Model with a catchy tagline: Everything we know – and don't know. His intellectual inspiration to delve into the slippery realm of the known-unknown is sourced from quotations (p. 1) of two key figures temporally distanced by centuries: Hippocrates and Winston Churchill. Both the quotations are instructive for us. Hippocrate's quote is: Life is short, the art is long, opportunity fleeting, experiment treacherous, judgement difficult. Churchill's is more governing-oriented, arising out of the policy failure of the Allies to defend Singapore from the invasion by the Japanese forces during the Second World War: I ought to have known. My advisers ought to have known and I ought to have been told, and I ought to have asked. Then again, uncertainties are not of the same genre and business analysts (Makridakisa et al., 2009:795) distinguish between at least two main varieties: subway uncertainties and coconut uncertainties. The first refers to what can be quantified and modelled. and reasonably incorporated in probabilistic predictions that assume, for example, normally distributed forecasting errors. The other pertains to events that cannot be quantified and modelled, and also to rare and unique events that are simply hard to envision. My choice of the two pieces from the world of pure business analyses is deliberate. I intend to emphasise the point that contrary to the general idea that business analyses only celebrate certainty and leave no space for uncertainty it is found that on certain occasions they are ready to acknowledge the inevitability of the failure to visualise everything that is going to happen. This lies in direct contrast to the governance analyses in which, as we have seen, it is the assertion of certainty all the way. There is an element of mystery in governance analyses being so because generically governance accords the driver's position to the market logic and in more ways than one governance becomes business.

To come back to the real world of governing in the pandemic era, in a significant development, after a long castigation of the WHO and its contradictory and confusing signals, it was the turn of the beleaguered organisation to try to turn the tables towards governments. On 14 July 2020, its Director General, meeting reporters in the aftermath of a record number of registered cases of 230,000 in 24 hours, chastised (News, 2020:1–13) a number of governments of the world for eroding public trust by sending 'mixed messages' on the coronavirus and neglecting public health to an alarming extent. He also warned that their failure to stop the spiralling outbreak means that there would be no return to the normal in 'foreseeable future'. Though he did not specify any country and qualified his statement with the comment that the economic, social and cultural consequences of lockdowns were creating problems for governments his observations – that 'too many countries are headed in the wrong direction' and that the power of the 'public enemy no.1' is not being matched by the actions it deserves and so it is 'going to get worse and worse and worse'— tell the tale quite adequately. It also reveals that if one major conduit of global governance, the WHO, is yet to convince the world about its efficiency the national governments are also in the same boat. It is also important that the WHO chief's admonition indicates that trust deficit and miscommunication are part and parcel of what many governments are doing. There is no prize for guessing that the two leading cases in this context would be the United States and Brazil even though they are not the only ones. It also substantiates our stance, stated already, that insofar as governing is concerned communication beyond its technological form, as meaningful social interactions created by exchanges of messages, data, information, experiences, interpretations, concerns and perspectives among policymakers, experts, stakeholders and public, has a crucial role. In his classic works, *The Nerves of Government: Models of Political Communication and Control* (Deutsch, 1963), much before the coming of governance with much fanfare, Karl Deutsch had explained innovatively how 'government' has communication channels as 'nerves'. In the days of governance as 'steering', as stated by its advocates themselves, Deutsch's term has come to be all the more important though in a more nuanced way than what he could depict by the largely technocratic cybernetic modelling. However, when it concerns governance communication a problem can be traced there too. By comparison, it gets less attention in the theoretical domain of governance, but even in the existing governance, where it has an inevitable presence, it surfaces more in the form of surveillance, miscommunication, false communication, rumour, fake news and so forth. In another book (Sinha, 2018:33–57) I have analysed in detail the importance of the communicative dialectics of governing, including the importance of governance communication as 'purposive connect' – in the backdrop of the shifting/sifting terms of governance in the contemporary times. In the analysis there has been an affirmation that governance, unmindful of the essential role of human-sourced *connections* and obsessed with the network-sourced *connectivity*, is more of a rhetorical exercise. The following chapters in this book contain deeper analysis of the communicative dynamics of governance in the same spirit from the specific vantage point of the COVID-19 pandemic.

To return to our main thematic concern, if one considers the basic framework of governing pandemic in a concrete way there are eight possible guidelines (Pandemic Response Report, 2009): i) Role Clarity – pandemic governance stakeholders must understand their respective roles during a pandemic response to foster informed decisions and timely action; ii) Level of Authority – the pandemic governance model must ensure that appropriate authorities exist to make key decisions during a public health emergency (for example, authorisation of emergency funding, performing emergency powers etc.); iii) Timeliness – the pandemic governance model must have the flexibility and capacity to allow for timely decision-making, dissemination of information and action to ensure that the government's essential services remain in operation; iv) Access to Subject Matter Experts – the pandemic governance model must have the ability to engage subject matter experts as needed (e.g., medical expertise) to provide critical information to decision makers; v) Coordinated Response – the government should ensure that the appropriate communication channels are in place during a pandemic emergency to allow for a timely and effective information flow and a coordinated effort across all stakeholder groups; vi) Succession Planning – government should ensure that a succession plan is developed and maintained for executive; vii) Knowledge Workers – all ministries and agencies must have an active cross-training programme in support of critical functions that require specialty knowledge; viii) Alignment – the framework should align and complement existing planning mechanisms and processes. Admittedly the above scheme has to be processed through multiple layers and perspectives not only of the administration but of the society and policy as a whole. The fundamental problem, however, arises when there is no clarity in the very first guideline, that is, role clarity. Role clarity calls for a clearer understanding of the interplay of the known and the unknown. It is to be built on the idea that 'clarity' does not necessarily entail cent percent certainty about what is to be done. It requires a fair degree of readiness to come to terms with the fact that various new factors would emerge in course of time and not all of them can be envisaged and forecast. But as I repeatedly mention, the coronavirus pandemic has shown a pathetic lack of role clarity on the part of almost all governments of the world. The super-criterion of efficiency as propounded by the exponents of good governance confronted COVID-19 and came to reveal an embarrassingly huge gap between role performance and role expectations in the governance agenda. The performance of governments vis-à-vis pandemic management has sought to be measured in course of time. Thus, the Sydney-based Lowi Institute has constructed a COVID-19 Performance Index (Lowi Institute, 2021), based on a 36-week study of 98 countries. The Index measures and ranks the countries in terms of their response to the pandemic with the exception of China because of the country's lack of public communication about its testing rates. New Zealand is ranked first, followed by Vietnam, Taiwan, Thailand and Cyprus. In contrast, Brazil is ranked among the lowest, with US being the fifth last. India is slightly higher with a rank of 86, a little above Bangladesh's 84th rank, but much below Pakistan's 69th and Nepal's 70th. Sri Lanka is the best performer in South Asia with a rank of 10. It is apparent that smaller countries have shown better performance and better performers are not necessarily economically sound. But what remains to be mentioned is that a major finding of the study is that leadership, irrespective of the political regimes, has also played a crucial role in determining the effectiveness of state responses. The study also mentions that the wider availability of vaccines may provide comparative advantage to the developed states in the time to come but till the middle of March of 2021 the findings are what they are. In this context one may add that while accusing 'authoritarian' China for failing to manage the pandemic (for whatever reasons) it is also important to analyse what ailed the management strategies of countries with political systems based on proclaimed 'democratic' governance. The countries had adopted the neoliberal development path with much aspiration but coming face to face with the pandemic they are left to fend for themselves Thus they have much to rethink about.

The global solidarity, a recurring promise in the governance agenda, especially in its advocacy of global governance, has been found to be wanting. One of the foundational claims of governance is the association and collaboration of civil society organisations and encouragement to public consultation in a systematic and regular manner. But the pandemic administration seems to have escaped such possibility. A survey (UHC Report, 2020) based on the analysis of 24 national COVID-19 Taskforces from different regions of the world reflects a very unhappy scenario. Its focus on the composition of the decision-making forces reveals that overwhelmingly the members are male politicians, virologists and epidemiologists, with very poor female and non-health experts. There is no representation of social workers, mental health experts, child health and development specialists, experts on chronic diseases or preventative medicine and human rights lawyers. It is found that if these types of experts were consulted at all, it was mainly as an afterthought. Except in few countries the civil society organisations have been kept at bay in the decision-making mechanism. One hundred and seventy five organisations responded to the survey and pointed out that their efforts were independent of their respective governments. Another important finding in the survey is that there is little transparency about whom the Taskforces are consulting. It is found that the evidence on which decisions are being made seems to be scientific and research-based from academic institutions, rather than drawing on from the lived realities of those groups most negatively affected by isolation and restrictive measures. In some cases the Taskforces comprise only government members, that too with the likelihood of participation from only education, interior and finance ministries. Ringing an alarm bell the report concludes that the societal consequences of isolation and lockdown measures are being overlooked in government decision-making and people, and that professions and organisations with potential for making meaningful contributions to the national response to the pandemic are simply not involved.

The pandemic caught the states on the wrong foot at a time when collaborations among them – often being vigorously defended by the emerging sub-domain of collaborative governance – was facing a very strained situation. It has been most evident in recent times with regard to the climate change issue. The inertia of the world leaders in this respect has led to a blisteringly critical speech by the Swedish teenage climate activist, Greta Thunberg. Her speech in the United Nations Summit on Climate Change included a stern rebuke – 'we will never forgive you' – to the leaders for what she regarded as a betrayal of young people. The way she was mocked by Donald Trump only exposes the failure of the governancing practitioners to respond constructively. During the pandemic, with some minimal exceptions here and there, it was clear that each country preferred to act in a standalone way. Be it in the countries in Europe or be it in those of the America and in the Indian subcontinent there has been little credible evidence of collaborative governance in the face of the emergency situation. Nor is there any substantial concrete evidence of the 'global civil society' acting in the collective spirit – something the global governance advocates, while justifying its overarching regulatory mechanisms for crisis management in a collective and cohesive manner, ceaselessly espouse as a foundational attribute. That all is not well with global governance is evident in a report (Hafner et al., 2020) on vaccine nationalism, a situation in which countries push hard to get first access to the supply of vaccines, potentially hoarding key components for vaccine production. The report projects that it might not only lead to the unequal allocation of COVID-19 vaccines but also would cost the global economy up to $1.2 trillion a year in GDP terms. The report also mentions (p. 1) that 'nationalistic behaviour' – marked by calls for nationalism in relation to the allocation of potential coronavirus vaccines, and by pressure on national governments to put their own citizens first – is inevitable even if there is adequate economic incentives for the high income countries like the USA, UK, and the European Union (EU) to provide vaccines to the low income countries. It specifically notes the possibility of global competition preventing the vaccine from reaching those who need it most and refers to lack of global cooperation as a plausible counterpoint to vaccine nationalism. It can be asserted that the pandemic has been quite efficient in a tweaked way in displaying that collective solidarity is still at a nascent stage.

The unbearable lightness of it all

Let me revert to the conceptual-theoretical mode of 'governance'. It seems that a major problem with the concept of (good) governance and its very constitutive logic is in its top-heavy character. When it was detached from the concept of government it not only sought to undermine the role of the (nation) state and underline the importance of the market as a mover and shaker of development. In the process it also detached itself from the formal institutional processes of collective action which lie at the core of the concept of government and the act of governing inscribed in it. It is not that in terms of its actual performance the government thesis was great, certainly not with the monopoly power enjoyed by the state. But the point is when the governance advocates go on to promise a much better mode, that too accusing the state of not adopting a sharing attitude in the decision-making process it was expected that in the days of governance things will be different. But is it not so? There is more to the intricate politics of governance than meets the eye – the contention may be clarified by referring to the theoretical formulations of governance by Gerry Stoker in one of the earliest and most read pieces.

Stoker provides (1998:18) five main propositions of governance: a) it refers to a set of institutions and actors that are drawn from but also beyond government; b) it identifies the blurring of boundaries and responsibilities for tackling social and economic issues; c) it identifies the power dependence involved in the relationships between institutions involved in collective action; d) it is about autonomous self-governing networks of actors; e) it recognises the capacity to get things done, which does not rest on the power of government to command or use its authority. Far from being contradictory or even competitive the propositions are complementary. Yet, he hastens to point out that there are certain specific dilemmas or critical issues associated with them. They are the following: i) a divorce between the complex reality of decision-making associated with governance and the normative codes used to explain and justify government; ii) blurring of responsibilities can lead to blame avoidance or scapegoating; iii) power dependence exacerbating the problem of unintended consequences for government; iv) emergence of self-governing networks raises difficulties over accountability; v) even where governments operate in a flexible way to steer collective action governance failure may occur. Stoker is sure that 'governance' is not detached from 'government' as it is only a developed or reinvented and better managed form with new tools and techniques, but with the same outcomes, the only difference lying in the adopted process. As he goes on to explain, the governance perspective in part builds on the challenge to the legal/constitutional tradition which lies at the conceptualisation 'government', but he also admits that it is not yet a smooth sailing process. Thus, in broadly challenging the conventional assumptions which focus on government as if it were a 'standalone' institution divorced from wider societal forces there is 'confusion and uncertainty' revealing the very first dilemma of governance.

Writing at the end of the twentieth century Stoker discovers the roots in the 'divorce' between the normative codes which are used to explain and justify government, and the reality of the decision-making process in the system, leading to tensions. He puts the onus on others for causing such inconvenience to conducting governance smoothly when he states that the public and more specifically the media lack a legitimation framework in which to place the emerging system of governance. He further defends the cause of governance by arguing that within any political system it is natural to have some ambiguity about rules and there will inevitably be some who do not accept their validity and who will not give their consent to the powerholders. However, he finds a lag in governance, lacking as it does the simplifying legitimising 'myths' of traditional perspectives, such as the British Westminster model, and observes that whether or how governance can obtain enhanced legitimacy is an issue worth considering. My point is that more than two decades have passed since Stoker made these observations, but governance is still short of the desired scale of legitimacy beyond what is lent by its theoretical advocates and practising power holders. But it is only a prelude to what can be regarded as a sweep vis-à-vis the crisis of governance, as evident in his observation on the fallout of the 'blurring of responsibilities'. He states (p. 21) that it creates 'an ambiguity and uncertainty in the minds of policymakers and public about who is responsible and can lead to government actors passing off responsibility to privatised providers when things go wrong. Worse still is the enhanced possibility of scapegoating raised by more complex governance systems. Those in a position to interpret and lead public debate can, often with considerable effectiveness, blame others for failures and difficulties. Blame avoidance and scapegoating are not new political phenomena, but governance structures do extend the capacity for such activity'.

On the sensitive issue of accountability, which has come under scrutiny in the pandemic era, Stoker visualises a problem. It is evident in his contention (p. 23) that the problem will arise as the self-governing networks are to a degree exclusive and are driven by the self-interest of members 'rather than a wider concern with the public interest or more particularly those excluded from the network'. This he observes even after emphasising (p. 22) that governance as an interactive process and multilevel partnership of self-governing networks implies a greater willingness to cope with uncertainty and open-endedness on the part of policymakers. Then comes the most significant idea of bringing government back in, with inculcation of 'appropriate codes' of governance, to achieve the goal of managing governance affairs by steering its much-celebrated networks. But even the lessons in 'appropriate codes' provide no guarantee of governance success. Stoker's final stroke lies in the clear acknowledgement (p. 24) that governance failure is 'crucial to the understanding of the world of governing'. This he describes as the paradox of the governance perspective. He traces the root causes of failure in tensions and difficulties with the institutions of civil society, inadequacies in organisations bridging the gaps between public, private and voluntary sectors, failures of leadership, differences in time scale and horizons among key partners, and in the depth of social conflict. The list seems to contain all the probable causes of failure of any system or order. Stoker makes it clear that he is not advocating governance while he analyses its perspective and problematises it. His epistemic orientation, as he himself notes, is more akin to the 'government in a governance' thesis (Kooiman and Van Vliet, 1993) than towards 'governing without government' as advocated by Rhodes (1996).

In another instance, this time writing with a co-author he argues (Pierre and Stoker, 2000:29) in this vein:

> The role of the *government* in the process of governance is much more contingent. Local, regional, national political elites alike seek to forge coalitions with private businesses, voluntary associations and other societal actors to mobilise resources across the public-private border in order to enhance their chances of guiding society towards politically defined goals.

However, after making some kind of see-saw movement vis-à-vis the idea of governance the comment (p. 25) one finds at the end of the article is that there is no turning back to the past, which implies that the government days and the changing world need to be studied as they are. The flexible spirit regarding the state comes back in the theory of metagovernance, which came into existence in the new millennium. It was the later phase of governance theorising to highlight the role of the state both in structural and social forms in coordinating mechanisms of governance and in steering the informal modes in complete collaboration with non-state actors. In the face of governance failure which was becoming gradually evident the idea was that the state would be vested with the task of coordinating various institutions – private, public and voluntary – without having any scope to assume the preponderant role that it had in the past. Those were the days of imagining 'governance without government'. Within a decade a new and revised perspective emerged. The coordinator in the new scenario is supposed to be the 'stateless state' (Bevir and Rhodes, 2011:203–217), also described as the 'hands-on state' with decentred design and approach, or in a more philosophical manner the state as 'meaning-in-action' – the social construction of patterns of rule through the ability of individuals to create meanings in action. Moreover, the institutions of the state generate contingent meanings that inform the actions of the individuals involved in all kinds of practices of rule. The approach has its obvious roots in the interpretive theory. The importance of the roots is clarified by Bevir (2010:3) with an attempt to associate it with postmodernism (though his neat adherence to certain formulations indicates otherwise) when he argues that interpretive social science certainly shifts our perspective on the relationship of knowledge to the state. He finds the shift in the process of moving away from the modernist social science's focus on how theories analyse the state to a broader look about how social science partly constitutes the state. Bevir raises much optimism about the possible link of the idea and reality of governance, especially in its democratic governance avatar, when he advocates the role of interpretive theory in this regard. As he writes (Bevir, 2010:266):

> An interpretive social science based on recognition of local reasoning typically leads to decentering, where to decenter is to analyze a practice in terms of the disparate beliefs of the actors. Interpretive social science concentrates on intentionality and so the meaningful nature of social life. Local reasoning draws attention to a creative if situated agency that suggests the beliefs or meanings held by any group, and even the ways in which they experience the world, are likely to be diverse and contested. Decentering thus consists in showing how an apparently monolithic institution actually embodies diverse, contested webs of belief informed by different traditions.

On the specific contribution of the interpretive theory in churning the notion of governance he (Bevir, 2010:58) notes the attempts by the interpretative theorists to resist the tendency to reduce governance and changes in it to allegedly fixed properties of systems, capitalism, institutions or rationality. He describes this as a manifestation of the 'legacy of mistaken positivism' encouraging social scientists to 'elide contingency behind allegedly objective social categories'. But a year later one finds a high dose of optimism about theory-practice complementarity somewhat moderated when Bevir and Rhodes (2011:210–211) refer to the under-performance of governance in carrying out in fulfilling its potential. In their defence they argue that their definition of governance pertains to a series of family resemblances that 'does not crave generality and aspire to comprehensiveness' because none of the resemblances need be always present.

Situating ourselves outside the analytic orbit of Bevir and Rhodes a deeper probe reveals that the decentred approach perfectly illustrates how a certain strategisation of flexibility, with open acknowledgement of the limitations of governance, creates a suitable template for its survival in the face of its evident failure in practice. Realising that notwithstanding much noise created around the cutting-edge concepts of 'metagovernance' and 'network governance' there still remains credibility deficit, the approach explains the 'shifting patterns' of governance by focusing on the actors' own interpretations of their actions and practices. It encourages flexibility by exploring the diverse ways in which situated agents change the boundaries of state and civil society by constantly remaking practices as their beliefs change. The approach rules out the measurement of governance by its key attributes. Thus, one cannot, if one adheres to the approach, critique the non-performance or under-performance of governance by referring to the attributes provided by the World Bank and the UNDP. The approach also insists that no attribute would be common to all the cases, thereby also negating the possibility of describing any particular case as a typical case of governance, the logic being that it is 'futile to search for the essential features of an abstract category that denotes a cluster of human practices' (Bevir and Rhodes, p. 211). This is how the flexibility imparts the 'lightness of being' in governance – in both theoretical and practical domains.

Whatever may be the politics of the stateless state thesis there is no doubt that the state has proved to have remarkable resilience of its own. The resilience may be a manifestation of its broader strategic manoeuvring, and not just of governancing. In rethinking governance from the other end of the spectrum Bell and Hindmoor (2009) contend that one main problem with the governance studies is that it does not recognise the possibility of modern states themselves mixing governance modes and even devising governance strategies in problem-solving acts in the policy domain. If this is true even to some extent it is indeed an interesting development in the sense that governancing is not just being infiltrated but configured by the new strategies of the state, an entity which is supposed to be at best its facilitator. To what extent, as these scholars' central claim goes, the state occupying a central position in modern society remains the major player in shaping and managing public governance, is subject to debates. But there are some notable empirical evidence of the state being brought back to salvage governing. Two strong advocates of the state refer (Olsen and Zamora, 2020) to Spain's requisition of private hospitals and medicine suppliers, Italy's renationalisation of its airliner Alitalia and that of the railways in UK, and Germany's plan to enunciate nationalisation by re-localising supply chains in sensitive areas. To them these are instances of the 'stunning turnaround' and the 'rediscovery of the state' as an instrument not only well suited to upholding a market order by enforcing competition and keeping public expenses at a minimum but also being able to boost the economy through fiscal policies and strong political measures for the common good. One may have issues with them regarding the claim that these trends are 'political alternatives' but there is no doubt that such developments reveal a change that was not thought of when the (good) governance thesis arrived with an aggressively hostile stance towards the state in the late 1980s and early 1990s.

It is revealing that when one Google searches 'governance failure' a huge number of entries come up on 'corporate governance failure' and some on 'government failure'. The search yields no result on the failure of 'governance' as the dominant system in the globalising world. It perhaps conveys the implicit messages that there can be no failure as such of the governance paradigm itself and if at all any reference to failure has to be made it may only be related to only one segment. It is true that even when there is an outpouring of literature examining governance from various vantage points during the occurrence of the COVID-19 pandemic the critical literature overwhelmingly, if not totally, emerges from those scholars, who are opposed to 'governance' tooth and nail. Such literature in most cases adopts an ideologically uncompromising stance and vociferously advocates the abolition of this genre of governance from the domain of governing, better still from the face of the earth, if possible. The other kind of 'critical' literature deals with possible shuffling and in some cases strategic reframing of private firms and multiple players of the corporate world, such as, shareholders, management, boards of directors, employees, customers, financial institutions and regulators.

I have already referred to the concept of 'failed state'. To refer to it more elaborately, the concept emerged in the politically significant 1990s and also became relatable to 'fragile states' which came up in the new millennium to connote the negative branding of the African states. These states became the 'perfect targets' for not being in league with the fixed terms of reference of aid by the Western donors. Deconstructing the 'failed state' discourse and highlighting the politics of political instability and extreme poverty Thiessen (2015:129–139) refers to the 'ambiguous, one-dimensional and self-serving' character, with the incontestable West-centric vision as the foundation. It is mentioned that the states are perceived as functioning entities and legitimate actors only when they pay the required obeisance to the donor assistance standards or to conditions set by the 'worthy states'. The notion that states can be divided into worthy and failed stems from the assumption, as Boas and Jennings argue (quoted in Thiessen, 2015:136), that 'all states can and should function in essentially the same way, and can therefore be located on a spectrum from good to bad'. On similar lines an insightful critique relating good governance and state failure was presented by Jones (2013), which prefers to situate the two concepts in the genealogies of the imperialist discourse. It knocks straight on the door of knowledge politics, with direct references to African Studies scholar Siba N'Zatioula Grovogui's critically acclaimed phrase 'racialised international knowledge' and his espousal of the ontology of difference. The core point in such (geo) political knowledge construction is the act of othering in which the underdevelopment of a country is solely the result of its own faulty path and that the chaos and anarchy in it are natural. Grovogui (2001) underlines the point that that the apparent empirical precision and objectivity of the analyses of state failure in Africa, though apparently shorn of the language of race, embodies a racialised imagination of European or western imperialism. Jones is right in asserting that like the state failure thesis the good governance thesis also presents itself as authoritative knowledge and becomes part of the common sense which depicts the African states as failures because of their inability to follow a particular line of development. Good governance, Jones agrees, is an attractive proposition if one goes by its very nomenclature and key attributes. But he expresses concern (p. 63) about its deceptive nature which, according to him, only apparently suggests a more positive approach than the conventionally pathologising diagnoses of fragility and failure, and in actuality it retains the essential form, structure and method employed faithfully mirrors that of the failure indexes. He clarifies that in analysing knowledge politics he consciously avoids confirming any direct relationship between the practices of global finance and the construction of failed states indexes even though they might form one component of information in the calculation of national credit ratings. Jones' suggestion is that the increasingly normalised use of indexes and rankings as a mode of producing comparative international knowledge, which is packaged in an apparently neutral and objective analysis of the capacity to govern and the risk of failure, might be located in the era of the hegemony of free market and global finance.

One may iterate that such search engine-based finding is a potent indicator of the dominant mode of knowledge politics that pervades the contemporary era. To put it succinctly, it stipulates that insofar as the actually existing governance is concerned there is no scope to contest, let alone refute, its parameters and to question its basic motive. There can at best be tinkering with some of its sub-sets ('corporate', 'private', 'environmental', 'multilevel', 'collaborative', 'adaptive', 'network'/'digital', 'platform' and so forth) but any anti-foundational, non-reductionist venture, which seeks to shake its discursive and empirical bases is ruled out. Having claimed complete grasp over knowledge of running the world it has a near-perfect command over what is to be done and how, thereby precluding any external forces from offering constructive criticisms of the mega-modes of governance. The periodic inclusion of prefixes such as 'good' and 'democratic' are the results of the underlying premise that the internal restructuring of the governance paradigm is more than enough to negotiate with the challenges of the times. Amidst the conceptual discussion it may be fruitful to refer to a medical anthropological case study of immense significance as far as the knowledge politics of governance is concerned. An ethnographic study by Leach and Tadros (2014) focuses on Egypt's contested narratives in H1N1 (the Swine Flu) response during 2009–2011, with reference to global health governance and biosecurity. It reveals, in a similar vein stated above, how particular kinds of knowledge and specific ways of knowing are co-constructed with the political positions and interests of particular actors. It also reveals how in the contexts of politics and power some streams of knowledge are privileged and deployed while others are suppressed or dismissed – with devastating results. In this case, H1N1 was represented as a pandemic and global security threat, justifying massive global response including the large-scale mobilisation of vaccines and antivirals. The WHO's role, as in the case of the coronavirus pandemic also came under cloud and it is stated that it was challenged and forced to justify its position. But the essay reflects a broader social concern which has relevance for understanding the dynamics of community engagement, an important component of pandemic management, to be discussed in Chapter 4. It does not require much effort to understand that this case is not the only one of its kind. An interesting study (Siedel and Vidal, 1997) of the HIV/AIDS policy in sub-Saharan Africa takes up the developmental and culturalist discourses HIV/AIDS and shows how each discourse is a particular 'way of thinking and arguing' about the epidemic and the reasons for its spread, which excludes other ways of thinking. What may be intellectual ferment for those who find in discourses a plausible source of democratisation the study notes that discourses – harbouring liberal doses of racism, sexism, stereotypes, metaphors, stigma among other factors and pushed by neoliberal meta-discourse – are not purely symbolic resources and arguments, but resources that may be politically invested by social actors, government or otherwise to achieve particular ends. The most striking result is the construction of Africa as an 'undifferentiated whole' incapable of change because of some immutable 'cultural traits' and 'cultural facts'.

In the case of policies emanating from the actually existing governance an essay (Siedel and Vidal, 1997:16) reveals that the language of policymaking seems to endorse realism. It is done by presenting 'problems', as if they could be solved by filling knowledge gaps with new objective, avoiding a language which says what is needed and by resting on descriptive accounts 'telling it as it is'. The domain of knowledge is neither a rigidly closed box nor is it complete and free from ignorance. The claim of (good) governance thesis bears on its shoulder the placard of 'good intention' and publicises its 'good will fund'. But those who have experienced the pinch, if not its blow, come to realise that behind such text there remains a contra subtext. The absence of preparedness for the unknown creates a filter in the actually existing governance, which in turn runs on an agenda based on a steep process of selection and exclusion. The domain of knowledge is neither a rigidly closed box nor is it complete and free from ignorance. The dominant narratives and associated pathways perform miserably in confronting the global pandemic because of their narrow instrumental aims sourced from such agenda. In a very interesting way another essay (Leach and Tadros, 2014: 240-254) reveals the intricate layers of politics of knowledge vis-a-vis the H1N1 epidemic. It concentrates on the suppression and delegitimisation of alternative narratives of the Zabaleen (Coptic Christians) within the borders of Egypt. It was done by branding a particular community as a 'ticking bomb' and 'diseased', and denigrating their lifestyle which depended much on pigs, as a source of imminent health hazard, namely, the plague. The irony of knowledge politics became evident when the legitimacy of pig culling resulted in aggravating the epidemic situation in total contrast to the expectations. The essay indicates the perverse manoeuvring of collaborative and multilevel forms of governance in the interest of the dominant forces in a particular setting.

In governance in normal times and more so in the pandemic times the adage 'ignorance is bliss' appears to carry dangerous portents. It is all the more dangerous if such ignorance is laced with hollow rhetoric. The refusal to recognise the unknown unknowns and then in the post-outbreak period the non-regocnition of the known unknowns lead to superficial blame games with the easy option of arbitrary, if not false identification, of risk group(s). It has also been proved that a denial mode regarding the existence and intensity of the pandemic, followed by an over-confident assertion that the existing knowledge based on the known knowns is more than sufficient to tackle the situation, puts the battle several steps backward. What has further complicated this situation is that the governments around the world have turned out to be more secretive when it comes to the disclosure of essential information about the pandemic. The attempt to hide behind rhetoric has not proved to be of any value. Thus, fixing the dates of the discovery of vaccine by political leaders and to put the responsibility of virus eradication on epidemiologists and biomedicine specialists also prove the hollowness of governing. It shows that those who boast of governance lack the faintest idea that the time path of discovery and the transformation of imprecise probabilistic predictions into precise probabilistic predictions involve many factors and social dynamics than just epidemiological and biomedicine knowledge and political compulsion. It also falsely equates fulfilling the official target date with the progress of science. Several warnings are being issued in this regard by concerned scientists and social scientists. It may be useful to mention some of them to provide an idea of their concern about rushing things in. In a commentary in *Science*, titled 'Against Pandemic Research Exceptionalism', two scientists (London and Kimmelman, 2020) identify the problem of 'deluge of clinical studies' marked by a sense of urgency and justifiably note that rather than generating low-quality investigations the urgency and scarcity of pandemics heighten the responsibility of key actors in the research enterprise to coordinate their activities to uphold the standards necessary to advance this mission. They call for balancing scientific rigour against speed on the ground that challenges that rigorous methods address do not disappear in the face of urgent need. One econometrician (Manski, 2020), a specialist in pandemic modelling, warns the researchers who might be falling victims to the rush syndrome that the tendency to replace uncertainty with 'incredible certitude' will only ensure pitfalls which are to be avoided at all costs. On another occasion he (Manski, 2020b) states that the credibility of the existing epidemiological models is still very limited and explains the futility of strategising mitigation and suppression of COVID-19 without ethical and economic implications. Noting the rise of conspiratorial theories in the coronavirus pandemic days, which even castigates Bill Gates for collaborating with the Chinese to benefit from the so-called Big Pharma, Epstein (2020) calls for paying serious attention to studies as part of the investigation of the politics of knowledge in COVID times. Having already convincingly demonstrated in a book (Epstein, 1996) how politics of knowledge works to reduce 'impure science' in the context of the AIDS he is suitably qualified to make such a plea. Expressing serious misgivings about scientists as vaccine researchers being trapped by the demands of the poor leadership one analyst (Cissé, 2020) traces the source of the problem in the 'always difficult but too often poor collaboration between scientists and policymakers'. In identifying a break between informed scientific policy advice and policy he does not find much difference between countries having different political systems, such as between China and France and USA. He also attributes the failure of global approaches to countering the pandemic to narrow nationalist responses and alarmingly bad policy decisions undermining the informed recommendations of scientists. Incidentally, a factsheet (Desikan et al., 2020:1–5) by the Union of Concerned Scientists in the US revealed how compared to the earlier epidemics the Trump administration took extra care to prevent public communication by scientists to ensure that public hear less from experts and more from leaders.

It is better to recognise that knowledge and ignorance are inseparable twins, not just in existential and empirical terms but also in ontological terms. Knowledge cannot acquire its value without referring to ignorance and that is precisely why it is linked to empowerment, and ignorance to disempowerment. But there is a catch, which should not go unnoticed. What is publicised as ignorance and regarded as so in the common perception may itself be the knowledge denied due recognition by the powers that be. Ignorance may well be delegitimated knowledge. In this sense 'knowledge is power' but the power emanates from some kind of coercion and exclusion, substantive and/or symbolic, through which certain specific ontological, epistemological, conceptual–theoretical and empirical varieties receive certification. The further the reach of the certification, the greater is the reliance on the known knowns at the expense of exploration of the known unknowns. Not just that, the neglect of the possibility of occurrence of unknown unknowns in foreseeable future also strengthens the false divide between knowledge and ignorance. Sir Francis Bacon had written 'knowledge is power' as the first line of 'Novum Organum', published in 1620. Later, how knowledge is put in the custody of the dominant forces has been most aptly expressed by Marx in *Critique of Hegel's Philosophy of Right* (1843) when referred to the 'baptism of knowledge' by the official recognition of the transubstantiation of profane into holy knowledge. The pioneering contribution of Pierre Bourdieu in enhancing our understanding of the role of knowledge in the form of cultural capital, as a conduit of diverse and subtle ways of perpetuating dominance of a particular social order, cannot but be acknowledged with all the appreciation it deserves. But leaving the well-known classical ideas for the time being one may refer to an emerging genre of studies on knowledge. It goes far behind to trace twists and turns in knowledge politics by hypothesising that the power of ignorance is basically a tactical ploy of domination – with the premise that 'ignorance' an act of giving meaning to a certain situation, not a given fact. It may have to wait for greater analytic purchase, but this is how in one instance the ethnographies of the power of ignorance are conceptualised (Doerr, 2009:293):

> What is new is our understanding that ignorance is not necessarily a cause and/or effect of being in the position of dominated in opposition to those with knowledge, but potentially a tool of the dominant to further reproduce the relations of dominance or to govern others and themselves in particular

> ways. Ignorance is an acknowledgement, which produces various readings of the situation, actions and effects that reflect, perpetuate, subvert or go beyond the given relations of dominance.

This game of ignorance may be played with some success until a catastrophic phenomenon like COVID-19 pandemic arrives and exposes it for all to see. When the field becomes too bumpy to play the game smoothly the inevitable question – at what cost the governance game continues – raises its head.

All these issues and questions are linked to pace. The neoliberal project rests on acceleration of everything under its tutelage. Speed thus becomes the spice of life and living, of survival, in the global times. Governance has to follow the same rhythm, otherwise it will lose its momentum. Thus, it has run so fast in its zeal to change the world according to the set rules of its parent ideology that it has left behind the vital issues of social security and individual and collective safety on the way. It has also undermined the logic that the domain of knowledge is neither a rigidly closed box nor is it free from ignorance. As a result, as mentioned earlier, there is a contradiction between the text and the subtext of governance. Take the example of network governance in this context. It is widely publicised for its association with democracy. However, the text has a subtext which reveals a much less positive scene when it comes to political equality, one of the core values of democracy. One cannot but notice the gradual descent of the realisation of the value in the practice of network governance, which is promoted as the hub of knowledge-based decision-making, creative problem solving and flexible well-coordinated policy implementation. The following excerpt (Dryzek, 2007:263) can be read in this context:

> 'Political equality' is on the face of it hard to operationalize in a network. Equality as an ideal is contested within democratic theory, but most conceptions of political equality define it in terms of citizens' proper positions in relation to the construction of sovereign authority: citizens stand formally equal before this authority, even if they are unequal in material endowments. Equality is a crucial aspect of democracy largely because individuals cannot easily exit the state; given that the state looms large and inescapable in the lives of members of the demos, the democratic ideal demands that they have equal capacity to influence what it does to them.... Networks generally do not loom so large, and it may be possible to escape the consequences of their decisions. Individuals can choose to exit networks in relatively costless fashion. They can less easily choose to exit the state, except by emigration and even if they turn their back on the state, it is likely to retain a very strong interest in them. Political equality as an ideal is less compelling in voluntary associations in which individuals are mostly only part-time participants.

The theme of political equality is chosen here for illustration because it is one of the ideals with profound significance for the process of social inclusion which faces erosion vis-à-vis governancing. It must be obvious that it does not mechanically mean direct participation of each and every citizen in the decision-making process. It means having fair representation of various segments of the society, including the underprivileged, in the existing political order. But the network governance is governed by the idea that with the networks providing enough autonomy to individuals there is no compulsive urge on the part of network managers to guarantee political equality in the way representative democracy, much critiqued by the governance advocates for its 'all round inefficiency', may provide. Networks often being issue-specific and informal at their core cannot be compared with the state when it comes to the degree of availability of opportunity for political equality. Dryzek is disarmingly candid when he poses the question whether the key (liberal) democratic ideals of popular control, political equality and rights to basic political liberties can be redeemed in the context of governance. His answer is unhesitatingly negative. Being one of the forceful advocates of discursive democracy he remains hopeful that such problem will be easier to work out and that governance networks can be democratised if the fit between such networks and 'talk-centric' deliberative, communicative approaches to democracy is given due attention. Then he notes that much remains to be done on this front, especially in translating the theoretical ideas into practice. Not just with network governance, even with discursive representation – which he continues to stoutly defend as a viable means to redeem the promise of deliberative democracy – he reveals in a co-authored essay (Dryzek and Niemeyer, 2008) that it itself is yet to solve many issues. The unsolved issues – including the possible modes, formal, informal or integrated-combined – fail to provide greater representation and be a sure-shot mechanism for deliberative democracy. So the knot remains, be it in the realm of governance or be it in its apparent redeemer, discursive democracy.

Migrant workforce: emblematic failing

One of the glaring instances of the under-performance of governance is the treatment meted out to the migrant workforce. The impact, both direct and indirect, of COVID-19 pandemic on migrant workforce, men and women (alongside the worsening conditions of displaced persons, refugees, students, children, the elderly, disabled, sex workers, LGBTQ) has been simply ruinous. It has engulfed the economic, demographic, political, social, cultural, logistic and administrative spheres in complex ways. The pandemic governance shed even the fig leaf of security and safety insofar as governancing migrant labour, primarily seen here as blue-collar workers and their families, is concerned. In contemporary times in which for many reasons social exclusion of the poor has been intensified and harshest measures introduced in the name of 'good governance' the migrants are bound to be the children of lesser gods in precarious existence.[2] Numerous pictures in media of the multitudes of dismissed wage labourers walking hundreds of miles to reach home, many falling ill and some losing life, testify to their dismal conditions. They are the highly dispensable element of the neoliberal regime and its instrument of governancing, especially in the realm of 'flexible' relations of production and distribution, and more specifically in the extremely exclusionary spectrum of labour, employment and work relations. The adverse conditions of the migrants around the world are certainly not a new phenomenon. But along with the outbreak of the pandemic it surely reached the lowest depth with a deadly combination of anxiety, panic, mental and physical illness, retrenchment/suspension from work, border closure and restrictions on movement by host and home countries alike. These measures are introduced, intensified and justified on the ground of public health but they have also resulted in allegations (Ramji-Nogales and Lang, 2020:593–602) that in the border closures the practice of restricting entry of the migrants and violating their rights the pandemic is being used as a 'convenient rationale' to enforce disproportionate disguising 'less salutary motivations' and 'unlawful political choices'. Significantly, the two most vociferous advocates of human rights and 'good governance', the USA and the EU, have come under heavy criticism in this regard. The EU deserves special mention in this context because of its claim of utmost concern with upholding labour rights.

'Coronationalism' has been intelligently coined to describe the zealous protection of borders in the name of 'national interest' during the pandemic situation. In this context a commentator (Trummer, 2020) explains with specific reference to the beleaguered East European caregivers in Austria that even the much vaunted supra-national entity like the EU was fragmented all of a sudden into 28 'national states' following policies of border closure as a result of the national borders being treated as the most important checkpoints for controlling the spread of the virus. It also leads the commentator to pertinently observe that COVID-19 has led to the revelation that the EU is a fragile construct that can easily get back into national state mode in times of serious trouble. The migrant labourers are also subject to stigmatisation and exclusion in ultra-nationalist, xenophobic and racist ambience – their insecurity and isolation reaching an abysmal point. For the governing establishment around the world – be it in the case of international migration the host/transit/countries of origin or be it the regions within the borders in the case of internal migration – migrants are supposed to remain stranded without basic amenities and even the right to life. Millions of nameless, faceless people, who are exploited by the growth engine of the economy in the normal times, are made destitute without any expectation of justice. It is only obvious that in such pandemic times, when governments of the world struggle with safety and security of their own citizens the migrant labourers would be the last to gain their attention, until and unless a section of them are found indispensable in some low-paid essential services. All the promises of social protection measures, packages and programmes, including those concerning decent wages, cash transfer, healthcare and health insurance coverage, have proved to be ineffective. A document (World Bank Brief, 2020) prepared by the World Bank Group, has the following observations (p. 6) to offer on the plight of the migrants:

> Lockdowns, travel bans and social distancing measures in response to the crisis have disproportionately affected internal migrant workers, who found

> themselves stranded, unable to return either to their places of work or their communities of origin. Without adequate access to housing, basic water and sanitation, health facilities or social safety nets to help them survive such restrictions, these migrants have become even more vulnerable to contagion risks. If discrimination and xenophobic attitudes affected migrants before, the current crisis has exacerbated such social tensions. The crisis has created a chaotic and painful process…

It may be mentioned that the World Bank itself is a major proponent of (good) governance. But if one goes through the list of suggestions mentioned (pp. 13–14) in the above-mentioned document one finds a tacit admission that not much has been done on any front to improve the situation of the migrants and with regard to their postponed or cancelled journeys. Beyond the emergency measures related to the coronavirus pandemic like the evacuation of stranded migrants and granting temporary protected status to foreign nationals with expired visas there is a call for serious attention to be paid to some short-, medium- and long-term strategies and measures such as health awareness campaigns, provisions of treatment and supporting informal businesses. There is also the mention of a host of other measures: grants to improve access to basic health services, education and housing, extending cash transfer programmes, providing incentives to reduce the cost of remittance services, revisiting the constraining insurance regulations, expanding origin countries' social welfare schemes to migrants abroad, facilitating the recognition of skills of migrants in host countries to help with the shortage of skills, supporting efforts to reduce remittance costs and achieving universal financial access in receiving and sending countries, supporting safe and regular migration programmes, supporting national strategies to increase the share of regular migrants in the total migrant population in host countries and establishing universal health programmes that include migrants irrespective of their legal status. The recommendations lay bare the stunted nature of economic and social security measures that were originally supposed to be the part of the migrant-friendly governance package.

Incidentally, noting how the 'age of accelerations' is also becoming an 'age of anger' another flagship document (World Migration Report, 2020) of the International Organisation for Migration also puts forth similar recommendations. But it does sot more exhaustively, combing the migration agenda with development agenda and global health agenda. Acknowledging the critical situation facing the actually existing governance it issues a warning note (p. 7):

> We are living in a period in which the core values underpinning global governance are being challenged. The values of equity, accountability, impartiality, fairness, justice and probity are being actively undermined as some political leaders disregard common interest in preference for personal interest – even if it corrodes laws, processes and institutions that have, overall, sought to advance whole nations and peoples, without excluding or expelling some

> because of their inherent characteristics or beliefs. Ongoing and systematic corrosion, as we have witnessed throughout history, can extend to attacks on human rights and ultimately on groups of people within societies.

Though the report was prepared before the outbreak of the current pandemic the excerpt provides valuable insights on the everyday functioning of governance in particular and the neoliberal ideology and rationality in general. In yet another report (Guadagno, 2020), prepared during the pandemic by the same organisation, that is, the International Organisation for Migration, there is an expression of grave concern about the vulnerability of migrants in access to healthcare, living conditions, work conditions and employment in different parts of the world. The three reports have a point of convergence in making it clear that when it concerns the formation of a stable and consensual framework of migration much remains to be done. But it goes without saying that nothing radically different would ever occur unless there is substantial change in the flexible production system and flexible labour market – the guiding force of such vulnerabilities – and constitutive elements of flexi-modernity. 'Contracting out', a valued instrument of the neoliberal regime, which is rationalised as an antidote to bureaucratism, has only aggravated insecurity in the employment sector by adding more and more people to the system and compelling them to take up temporary and/or casual work – with no occupational identity and security of their own. The irony is that any radical change in the exploitative system is going to be resisted at all costs by the neoliberal plutocracy.

Concluding remarks

Pace is welcome but governance-in-haste is a rule by denial, with the tagline 'divided we stand'. The rise of the precariat, including the migrants, and their plight during the coronavirus pandemic testify to the 'unbearable lightness' of governance from the ethical standpoint. In the very title of the chapter a question has been posed – lockdown or meltdown? The answer goes in favour of the former. The pandemic has not only brought in lockdown as a key administrative measure to restrict viral transmission but it has also put governance-in-practice under lockdown. Yet, as already noted on several occasions, governance has an exceptional survival instinct. It faces numerous dilemmas and crises but it does not reach the state of meltdown. In practice governance is going to remain the dominant mode of governing in the contemporary world. Its umbilical cord with the neoliberal project ensures its survival, with no feasible and sustainable alternative governing mode with as much power and reach in sight as yet. One may call it the not-so-strange non-death of governance. Taking the matter further the next chapter will discuss how governance not only survives but also seeks to consolidate its position with cutting-edge technology.

Notes

1 The following books, though only indicative, contain a large number of brief essays on governance and provide a fair idea of its spectrum and dynamism: Mark Bevir ed., *The Sage Handbook of Governance*, London: Sage Publications, 2011; David Levy-Faur ed., *The Oxford Handbook of Governance*, Oxford: Oxford University Press, 2012; Christopher Ansell and Jacob Torfing, *Handbook on Theories of Governance*, Cheltenham: Edward Elgar, 2016.

2 I am not rushing in to fix the migrants to the important yet controversial concept of 'precariat' formulated by Guy Standing in *The Precariat: The New Dangerous Class*, Bloomsbury: Bloomsbury Academic, 2011. The reason is that I am not too sure whether the migrants have reached a stage in which like the precariat they are increasingly able to identify what they wish to combat and what they want to construct, or to what extent, if at all, they have attained the class status. But at the same time, I find in Standing's formulation some important clues, especially, the villainisation of migrants and their fear and anger from a sense of deprivation, and also food for thought in the overall process of 'precariatisation' and the systematic insecurity it entails.

3

GOVERNANCE COMMUNICATION

The biopolitical trigger

Introduction

There are, and there should be, debates on the pros and cons of governance. As noted earlier, some zealous advocates of governance tend to find no fault with it, lesser number of its more serious votaries make efforts to firm up its conceptual-theoretical foundation for greater credibility, and some find it hopelessly incapable of ensuring a better world for most people. However, on one issue there is no disagreement at all among the advocates and adversaries – that neoliberalism constitutes its philosophical foundation. Once it is accepted by both sides it is only natural that governancing will be defended at all costs by its advocates even when its fault lines continue to be exposed, and even when they are laid wide open during the COVID-19 pandemic. By the same logic it is also obvious that the sponsors and promoters of governance will strike back with all the wherewithal at their disposal when confronted with such severely embarrassing situation. One of the best ways for them to do it is to utilise cutting-edge information and communication technologies (ICTs), which have incredible reach and penetration to regulate human life. Behind the public rhetoric of utilising the ICTs for public welfare one can trace efforts to utilise digital interconnectivity to intensify the paranoid obsession with surveillance through governance. The practice of algorithmic governmentality will be discussed extensively in Chapter 4. At this point, let me iterate that there is more to communication than the ICTs, and for this reason one needs to go beyond a crass instrumentalist approach to communication. One may venture to add that the pandemic-centred surveillance and the regimentation that conducts it is far more sophisticated than what George Orwell could depict in *1984*. The governments are the 'watchmen' no doubt, but the gamut of governance through regimentation is much more sophisticated and complex now. Having the advanced and finely tuned technology at their disposal, the sponsors of governancing are in

DOI: 10.4324/9781003247388-4

a better position to ensure conformity among the publics, and more so when it concerns the 'pandemic publics'. The subtle initiatives in no small measure are to be attributed to the refined process of 'normalisation', as distinct from crudely invasive techniques. Pandemic and the crisis it entailed as though automatically injected a strong dose of 'legitimation' to surveillance in the name of health protection. The situation entails disease detection, outbreak tracking, identification of vulnerable sections, preventive measures and so forth on a daily basis with very active intervention mode. The whole process also involves collection of a host of information about the population, including those of the most private nature, raising questions of the delicate balancing healthcare treatment and protection with individual rights. In some countries, including China, innovative technologies like artificial intelligence (AI), big data, drones, robotics, automated block chain and 5G are extensively used to ensure proactive interventions. The technological efficiency has taken a toll in reliability of data and democratic decision-making.

The most important point to note in this context is that the 'technologies of discipline' literally infiltrate the human body, and beyond the physicality of it all they also make mental impacts on the human 'hosts'. In this sense, the immersive technologies and coronavirus share a common operational mode. One can find the origin of such convergence, as does Peters (2012:98–111), in the broader political economy of new technology. The convergence is to be especially found in the give-and-take relations between biology and information and in the umbilical relations of bioinformatics and bioinformational capitalism, which ensure a hitherto unforeseen impact on life, including intensification of privatisation and monopolisation of knowledge. Alongside the role of the broader political economic development causing the proximity of 'bio' and technology, the impetus to 'bio' at this point in time has a disciplinary shuffle as well. Thus, a study (Peters et al., 2020) on the bioinformational paradigm of the coronavirus pandemic refers to the disciplinary resurgence of biology and the simultaneous fall of physics. The rise and fall are described as the cause and consequence of the interplay of bioinformational capitalism and knowledge capitalism. The study finds the reverberation of the process in the biologisation of the digital which follows the digitalisation of biology. The rise of biology is found in the larger size of its budgets, workforce and in the output of major discoveries – with economic, ethical consequences and welfare implications.

In this chapter, continuing from the previous chapter, I seek to explain how amidst its non-/under-performance during the pandemic times the governance-in-practice utilises the power of new technology and undermines what are supposed to be its own prime attributes – accountability, transparency and responsiveness in particular – and democracy in general. The discussion here has the main focus on the role of bioinformation, regarded as a major element of the disciplinary force of biopolitics, as a major mechanism of regime rationalisation and 'authoritative knowledge, for manoeuvring the known and the unknown. In such stance I shall follow the recent research trends in which bioinformation, beyond its still dominant nesting in science (especially genomics and bioinformatics), is related to the social, political and economic variables rooted in the contemporary neoliberal era. Also, in accordance with the thrust in this volume on the communicative dialectics of the issues concerned Foucault's classic statement (Foucault, 1995:200) on the mechanics of the Panoptican surveillance – that one remains the object of information but never a subject of communication – is kept in mind. Let me also add at the outset that a surveillant society is a dangerous proposition. It is much about reproducing the surveillance logics and making them inherent to social order. It may someday result in society being popularly imagined in a manner in which there is inscrutable affective attachment to modes and instruments of surveillance, and the surveillance acts becoming an integral part of people's identity. In this context the coronavirus pandemic may be treated as a 'dress rehearsal'.

Biopolitics: governing body

The focus here on biopolitics/biopower and on bioinformation and biocitizenship in the following section has a broader perspective: the coming together of 'governance' (to reiterate, as shaped in a specific historical juncture), and 'governmentality' as conceived originally by Foucault. That the discussion here devotes much more space to biopolitics/biopower and bioinformation should in no way be construed as the mark of reduced importance of governmentality. It is because they are its vehicles. The basic argument here is that with regard to the governance deficit in the ongoing calamitous times there is a clear indication that the intense securitisation measures based on regulating the life of population is sought to be sustained, at least in near future. The way the governments around the world are adopting, in the name of pandemic governance, the technique of control makes it evident that more than ever before governance and governmentality are coming closer – and too close for comfort.

Despite not being the same constructs and having different intellectual origins governance are governmentality are incorporating many common features and objectives as part of their collaborative undertaking. The pandemic has paradoxically provided an opportune moment to hide governancing deficiencies while exposing them. The adopted strategy in this context is the 'offence is the best defence', based on the intensification of specific protocols of governable, orderly and disciplined populations. The practicalities of it all also involve a deeper dimension – the dynamics between individualising technologies which are fundamental to the formation of subjectivities, and the totalising technologies aimed at populations as large collectivities. Like governance and governmentality, which are different yet closely connected, both varieties of technologies are not the same but are intimately linked. Foucault in *Discipline and Punish: The Birth of the Prison* (1995) laid a foundation on which governance and governmentality – their 'whys' and 'hows' – can be related. It can be done even at a time which would be different from his specific historical references. In situating them in the knowledge/power axes, which lie at the base of the known-unknown dialectics prioritised in our discussion, Foucault left some vital cues to realise, especially in these times, that governance is much more than a mere instrumental and mechanical mode of 'steering' and it is capable of aggressively transforming into 'conducting'. There is much truth in the observation (Burchell, Gordon and Miller, 1991:x) that the major contribution of the Foucault Effect lies in generating the awareness that the sense and object of governmental acts do not fall from the sky or emerge in ready form from social practice. They are things, as the argument goes, which had to be – and which have been – invented.

Yet biopolitics is an innovative but highly complex theme not just in governing but also in the conceptual domain. To begin with, both 'bio' and 'politics' defy easy definitions. The first is connected with life and living beings, but as 'bios' it relates to the more complicated issue of how life is lived. The other, that is 'politics', at least the way it is perceived here, is inextricably linked to power relations vis-à-vis the act of governing, involving the rulers and the ruled. Biopolitics keeps distance from both positions. Noting how the notion of biopolitics detaches itself from the naturalist and politicist approaches, both of which treat 'life' and 'politics' separately and fail to account for their relationality and historicity, Lemke (2011:4) explains how it signals a double negation:

> The impact of biotechnological innovations has demonstrated that life processes are transformable and controllable to an increasing degree, which renders obsolete any idea of an intact nature untouched by human action. Thus, nature can only be regarded as part of nature-society associations. At the same time, it has become clear that biopolitics also marks a significant transformation of politics. Life is not only the object of politics and external to political decision-making; it affects the core of politics—the political subject. Biopolitics is not the expression of a sovereign will but aims at the administration and regulation of life processes on the level of populations. It focuses on living beings rather than on legal subjects – or, to be more precise, it deals with legal subjects that are at the same time living beings.

To raise an important conceptual issue about biopolitics, it has an intimate link with biopower (Liesen and Walsh, 2012; Adams, 2017; Rainbow and Rose, 2006), particularly in the context of the Foucauldian framework of governmentality. Yet, Foucault did not gift us with crystal-clear meanings of the two key concepts as he continued with their slow and gradual mode of evolution. He has been criticised for keeping them half-formed and falling short of being radical to the extent expected from a thinker like him. One may also think of the possibility that he did not live long enough to fulfil his promise of writing a book on biopower. Or it may also be imagined that he had been exploring them in heuristic terms (even as 'teasers') to be adopted and developed further by other scholars, a practice which has indeed occurred and contributed to many studies critically reflecting on various metrics of the exercise of power. In the field of Political Science, which has power as its fundamental unit of analysis there are multiple and competing meanings of biopolitics. In course of time, one finds an analytical strand in which no extra effort is made to distinguish the two concepts. In my case the distinction between the two is acknowledged. Without delving into a deep genealogical exposition the discussion here treats biopolitics to be a genre of political rationality, entrenched in 'deadly form of power'. It treats the administration of life and populations as its subject with the avowed purpose of ensuring that life is 'orderly' – and considers biopower as its driving force.

Curating several works of repute on biopower Rainbow and Rose (2006:195–217) contend that the concept designates 'a plane of actuality' that must include, at a minimum, the following elements: First, one or more truth discourses, which may hybridise biological, demographic and even sociological styles of thought about the 'vital' character of living human beings, and an array of authorities considered competent to speak that truth. Second, strategies for intervention upon collective existence in the name of life and health, sometimes specified in terms of categories of race, ethnicity, gender or religion, as in the emerging forms of genetic or biological citizenship. Third, modes of subjectification, through which individuals are brought to work on themselves, under certain forms of authority, in relation truth discourses, by means of practices of the self, in the name of their own life or health, that of their family or some other collectivity, or indeed in the name of the life or health of the population as a whole. The biopolitical act is no less characterised by a steep gendered vision, in which women are often the special target. This has also led to the growth of the feminist perspectives (for instance, Corrêa, 2020) on a general scale and also in the specific context of the coronavirus pandemic. In the latter case of the biopolitical dimensions and impact of the pandemic efforts are made to develop a conceptual frame for better understanding of the centrality of gender, reproduction, sexuality and race in the complex assemblage of capitalism (as the economic formation), the sovereign nation state (as the 'only existing' polity model) and a vast web of administration and regulation disciplining life.

The complexities created by COVID-19 not only leads to ferments in the conceptual terrain of biopolitics it has even raised the possibility of recasting both 'bio' and 'politics' in new frames. Foucault had presented dreadful sovereigns of four centuries – from the seventeenth to the twentieth – since the 'threshold of biological modernity', who would leave no stone unturned in seizing, repressing and destroying life. But the way both 'bio' and 'power' come together in the post-Information Revolution era they turn out to be a concoction of developing, managing, optimising, ordering and securing life in both individual (self) and collective realms in a manner which would perhaps make the earlier instances pale in comparison. Foucault did an intellectual reverse sweep in making us aware that rather than 'bio' determining the contours of politics it is the other way round. Thus he writes (2013 [1976]:67):

> What we are dealing with in this new technology of power is not exactly society… nor is it the individual-as-body. It is a new body, a multiple body, a body with so many heads that, while they might not be infinite in number,

> cannot necessarily be counted. Biopolitics deals with the population, with the population as a political problem, as a problem that is at once scientific and political, as a biological problem and as power's problem.

The pandemic has reinvigorated his thesis of subjugation of body and control of population beyond any doubt, but it has done so with newer dimensions, angularities and techniques. It has confirmed the extended versions of biopolitics as espoused by Agamben, and Hardt and Negri. It has considerably renewed Hardt and Negri's reference (2009) to power regulating social life 'from its interior'. Agamben, notwithstanding his wrong estimation of the pandemic mentioned earlier, does have the satisfaction of witnessing how the pandemic tends to confirm his thesis of the 'state of exception' (2005) – taking advantage of the emergency situation and promulgating highly restrictive protocols of movement, mobility, services and activities of various kinds. In a later commentary on the pandemic, more profound than his first one, Agamben (2021) apprehends that with the pandemic times we are increasingly coming under 'government of the faceless and the deathless', with such registers as masks, social distancing and algorithm-based governmentality. Significantly for the discussion here, he specifically mentions how such phenomenon overplays (digital) information at the cost of (physical) communication. Thus, we find that be it Hardt and Negri or be it Agamben information and communication play a crucial role. I shall further complicate the relationship with the emerging concept of bioinformation. For my purpose in this section let me just briefly state that bioinformation is parented by biopolitics, and for that matter, by biopower too.

There is no attempt here to establish the point that the COVID-19 pandemic is the first of its kind to introduce bio-surveillance through releasing bioinformational modes. For instance, Parry (2012:718–725) finds solid evidence of the promulgation of new, more robust and finely calibrated systems of biological surveillance, facilitating the creation of new, expansive and very pervasive forms of governmentality, during the H1N1 (Swine Flu) pandemic in USA and UK. One can go even further back to find evidence in some earlier pandemics as well. But beyond doubt, the fine-tuning of the COVID-19 pandemic and the unending rattling of data and information coalescing body, population, race, ethnicity, birth, life expectancy, longevity, death, health, welfare, security, safety, morbidity, life expectance, survival, medicine, care, science and technology, clinical tests/trials, efficacy of vaccines and so forth have unleashed biopolitical surveillance – the control of populations by measuring, apprising, hierarchising population through apparatuses of normalisation in order to maximise life processes with unmatched spread and depth.

To resonate Foucault, the illness of a vast number of people and the crisis that followed led to the intervention of some by their kind of knowledge, resources and pity. But there is a need for inserting a qualifier here. Coronavirus has a much greater 'real time' impact than leprosy, plague and smallpox, the diseases which had primarily occupied Foucault's mind. It also has a much larger 'grey' frame of life and death, to borrow another important element from the Foucauldian framework of biopolitics, originally termed as anatomo-politics. In a bewilderingly fast strike the pandemic has engulfed the world in a way that has no other instance in history. As noted, the declaration of the disease as pandemic by the WHO has been a sort of blessing in disguise for governancing as it has opened up opportunities to reinstate acts, regulations and orders with the warnings of stringent punishment for defiance or disobedience. Considering the empirical evidence available there is no reason to believe that the states with 'firm' democratic polities were slower players in the race for establishing what Foucault would describe as the 'totally administered society'. The 'shared threat' almost instantly became 'shared surveillance' to such an extent that it would have perhaps surprised even Foucault, had he been alive today. Even if the somewhat misleading term 'social distancing' was not in vogue in Foucault's days what he classically depicted (1995:195; brackets mine) in *Discipline and Punish* in the context of plague rings astonishingly true: 'It is a segmented, immobile, frozen space. Each individual is fixed in his place. And, if he [sic] moves, he [sic] does so at the risk of his life, contagion or punishment.' Unlike Leonardo da Vinci, Foucault did not indulge in preparing a new blueprint for city governance, but what he had unravelled in terms of the intentions of the rulers is sure to hold relevance for a long time to come. The relevance concerns not just the restrictive acts of the rulers, but also in a metaphorical way their dream of an epidemic-like plague to coming to their aid to exert control over people through surveillance. Foucault's overarching idea of the disciplinary society through hierarchisation, normalisation and examination holds true despite the critical argument (Sarasin, 2020) that he went on modifying his ideas on the basis of three different ideal-typical models based on leprosy, plague and smallpox. Sarasin mentions that Foucault had distanced himself from the idea of biopolitics by the end of the 1970s, but asserts in the same breath that the analytic value of the idea remains intact. The works that follow Foucault's exposition of biopolitics in the mid-1970s reveal that its expiry date is not yet close even though it is bound to be subject to further extensions. Some such works will be discussed here but let me mention that even the most radical critique of the Foucauldian thesis of biopolitics/biopower, the one based on necropolitics/necropower, does not call for its negation. The necropolitical dimension was conceptually initialised in the context of war and sovereignty by Achille Mbembe (2003). Mbembe had found Foucault's (Eurocentric) explication of biopolitical management deficient at least on two counts: in having lack of understanding of the key role of colonial slavery and in falling short in referring to the state's extreme power over lives as manifested in categorising populations into 'useful' (who may live) and 'disposable' (who must die). In relating necropolitics and the 'repressed topographies of cruelty' to the functioning of capitalism in which everyone has a (market) price, and everything is weighed in terms of profit Mbembe raises (p. 12) a set of pertinent questions, which includes the following: i) Under what practical conditions is the right to kill, to allow to live or to expose to death exercised? ii) What place is given to life, death and the human body? iii) How are they inscribed in the order of power?

There is no doubt that the exploration of these questions in the context of the thoroughly inequitable and exclusionary coronavirus pandemic would take us a step further than the Foucauldian analysis in understanding how the vast populations are subjected to the 'conditions of life conferring upon them the status of living dead' (Mbembe, 2003:40). At the same time the necropolitical edifice having been built on the Foucauldian base contributes to enhancing the horizons of biopolitics/biopower. One may even hazard a guess that had Foucault been alive to see governance in such pandemic times he would have analysed biopolitics in novel ways. The ensuing discussion will shed some light on some such extensions of the original Foucauldian framework of biopolitics, which only prove the power of the original venture.

Foucault's relevance becomes all the more evident when one finds that even analysts (Hannah, Hutta and Schemann, 2020), who do not claim that the pandemic situation can be comprehensively explained by the Foucauldian methodological lens and analytical framework, assert that the contemporary scenario is an evidence of constellation of the Foucault-sourced elements of sovereignty, discipline, biopolitics/biopower, and governmentality, all of which combining and operating in uneven and rapidly shifting ways. Even in Foucault's absence there is a scope, as Sarasin (2020) himself reveals through four (transitional and overlapping) developments, based on the three infectious disease models, to relate one of the most influential ideas of our epoch to the coronavirus times. First, the complete lockdown of Wuhan rigorously follows the plague model, and every other curfew ultimately does the same. The imposition of curfew as a departure from the more liberal smallpox model is necessitated because there is inadequate statistical knowledge of the phenomenon. Sarasin also notes that only when systematic tests supply massive amounts of data about infected and non-infected people is it possible for governments to restrict themselves to isolating the infected and recommend caution for the rest of the population, without having to impose a lockdown. He cites the examples of South Korea and Singapore in this context, in which public life goes on and the economy continues to function without major glitches. Second, he describes the plague model as a threat, even as a danger. In this context he refers to the introduction of harsh military measures and the visuals of tanks in the streets of Morocco to impose curfew, the possibility of engineering a 'coup' in the name of countering the virus by the ruling regime in Israel, the plan of transition to a government by decree in Hungary and the effort of the US Attorney General to hold prisoners indefinitely without trial. Then he adds the 'knowledge dimension' in speculating that the storage and evaluation of movement data of everyone carrying a mobile phone is unlikely to be easily relegated to a purely technical possibility after this crisis. These trends, he also notes, are far removed from the liberal smallpox model which fundamentally and always requires that the power of the state be monitored with suspicion. Third, even while acknowledging differences and varieties of 'national egotism' he is quite indulgent to the European governments in associating the liberal smallpox model to their regimes. Sarasin specifically refers to the strategy of flattening the curve, which in his interpretation reckons with the pathogen on the understanding that it cannot be eradicated but its distribution can be extended over time to enable the health system to handle the crisis. On the strategy of prohibiting gatherings of several people he seems certain that it does not amount to 'discipline', but it is rather 'something like a narrow but well-justified and understandable framework' the state sets for individual behaviour. He goes on to provide almost a sweeping approval to the European governments in this regard by his argument that in general the call to observe rules of social distancing belongs 'without doubt' in the sphere of liberal techniques fundamentally based on individual freedom. The only call that he has for the European governments is that they must respect such freedom. He is also confident that the liberal smallpox model is effective in tackling the complex dynamic of the self and the community. As he observes:

> To take care of oneself, to protect oneself, but also, as can widely be observed at the moment, to find forms of neighbourly or solidary organisation are techniques of the self that fill the liberal contours of the smallpox model with the concrete material of social self-organisation.

Fourth, Sarasin is apprehensive that the leprosy model is lurking in the background, especially in such atrocious idea that let old people die to save the economy or in the factual reality when retirement homes and nursing homes are abandoned with inmates dying locked up and alone. It may be mentioned that the European governments are not totally immune from both the 'strategies'. The Italian government faced allegations during the outbreak that it was being neglectful of the elderly (though there was no solid evidence of any such systematic attempt). In Spain's case, as Sarasin himself mentions, the retirement homes and nursing homes had a fair number of lonely, abandoned inmates waiting to die. He has been a bit too generous about the attitude of the European governments and his stance has provoked criticism by various analysts – to be mentioned subsequently.

We may, despite being critical of his hasty assessment of the pandemic, for the time being distance ourselves from the call for 'saving the society from Agamben' and pay attention to Agamben's highly critical observations on the Italian government's alleged measures to counter the pandemic. Here too he may have some excesses but that does not negate his concern for the protection of rights and freedoms of the populations. As Agamben observes (2020b):

…the recent provisions (taken by the Italian government with decrees that we would like to hope – although this is nothing but an illusion – will not [sic] confirmed by parliament, and turned into laws) actually transform every individual into a potential infector, exactly as the laws on terrorism considered, de facto and de jure, every citizen to be a potential terrorist. The analogy is indeed so clear that the potential infector who does not comply with the prescriptions will be punished with prison. The figure of the healthy or unwitting carrier – who infects a multiplicity of individuals, unable to defend themselves from him, as one who defend oneself from the infector – is presented as being extremely sinister.

Even sadder than the curtailing of freedom implied by these measures is, in my opinion, the degeneration of the relationships between men [sic] endangered by them.... The other, whoever he may be, even a loved one, must not be approached or touched.... Our neighbour has been abolished.... (W)e stop encountering each other and to speak about politics or culture...

Agamben is not alone in expressing such sentiment. The same kind of apprehension is expressed not only from thinkers like him but also from the analysts from other domains of life. Introducing a new issue on the Index on Censorship, with the telling heading 'Private Lives: What Happens When Our Every Thought Goes Public', Rachael Jolley (2020:1–3) in an editorial note bemoans the fact that while on the one hand governments are reticent about informing the public about the pandemic they on the other hand are ramping up surveillance and cracking down on privacy. This way of taking away of basic freedoms of people in times of crisis, according to her, destroys the trust that government will not collect private information about citizens and will not use the collected information without informing them so essential in relations among the rulers and the ruled. Unlike Australia where legislations protect citizens from the use of personal data of citizens by government, in Britain (till the time of her writing) she notes (p.3) that there has been no sign of legislation outlining any restrictions on how data captured by its track and trace system, or expected COVID-19 app, will be restricted from other use, or even stopped from being sold to third parties. In the construction and analyses of the Index different resource persons identify four key areas in this process of transgression, much of which are propelled by the ICTs. The identified areas are:

i) New normal: contact-tracing apps can be effective in containing the pandemic, but they can also have unintended consequences. After the emergency, contact data may be of use to the police and government, not to mention advertisers who have immense influence in determining the construction of data. The argument is that in exceptional times we might have no option but to accept measures that would normally be considered draconian, but they must remain exceptional, and not become the new normal.
ii) Sexual privacy: Contact-tracing, legitimised by COVID-19 security risks, is already a dating app reality. This may take the lid off the privacy of LGBTQ communities and expose them to abuse, especially in countries in which they are treated with disdain.
iii) Facial recognition: The use of facial recognition technology is on the increase as governments seek to monitor the spread of the virus. But its effectiveness – often not scrutinised enough – needs to be weighed against the risks it poses to human rights. The identity may be sold commercially and thus may make victims out of unsuspecting individuals.
iv) Drones: Loudspeaker-equipped drones issuing safety warnings during the pandemic have been deployed in a number of countries. But the debate over how data protection law should apply is lagging behind. Noting that drones are

> being increasingly used even in Britain a question is posed whether in the post-lockdown restrictions they may be combined with facial recognition to track individuals.

The observation about Britain contests Sarasin's optimistic projections about the European countries. That Sarasin has a slightly faulty vision becomes apparent from a more acute observation (Hannah, Hutta and Schemann, 2020) that even in the cases of those states in Europe where total lockdown and the strict stay-at-home orders were not imposed the presence of the disciplinary power was evident. It is pointed out that dramatic reductions in public activity produced a 'background' against which those who are still present in public would stand out more clearly and could be required to justify their presence.

There is another vital dimension to the phenomenon of governmentality. It is not always the case that everything has to be necessarily imposed from above. The population may show 'impressive' degree of conformity in a number of cases. Thus, scholars like Lorenzini (2020) has a different take on the issue, quite a departure from that of Agamben's, that instead of worrying about the increasing surveillance mechanisms an indiscriminate control and the coming of a new 'state of exception' it might be prudent to worry about our already docile nature as 'obedient biopolitical subjects'. Ruminating on the nature of biopolitics in pandemic times Lorenzini comes close to the 'interior' dimension of biopolitics because he realises that the biopolitical power is not (only) exercised on our lives from the 'outside', as it were, but has been a part of what we are, of our historical form of subjectivity, for at least the past two centuries. In defining the 'political grammar of the crisis' he directly takes on Agamben and argues that Foucault's work on biopolitics is more complex, rich, and compelling during the time of coronavirus than what it appears to be under the pen of those who too quickly reduce it to a series of anathemas against disciplinary confinement and mass surveillance or who misleadingly utilise it to talk about the state of exception and bare life.

I shall come back to this point and relate it to what is being theorised as 'populist biopower'. Let me add that Lorenzini has another interesting point to add to the analysis of biopolitics in pandemic times: his formulation of the (bio)politics of differential vulnerability. Though he has his main focus on the relationship between biopower and race in the formulation – in the process bringing in Butler, Nancy and Latour into the debate – what comes out from his arguments has broader relevance in critical social thinking. To him, it is that kind of politics which structurally relies on the establishment of hierarchies in the value of lives, producing and multiplying vulnerability as a means of governing people. Lorenzini refers to the newfound practice of collectively applauding the medical heroes and care workers, the frontline personnel in the fight against the virus. But even when he acknowledges their role in this regard, he questions why other categories of people serving us directly during quarantine and risking their lives – the supermarket and pharmacy cashiers, public-transportation drivers, factory workers, police officers – are not being considered 'care workers'. In this argument he goes against the description of coronavirus as a 'great equaliser' and provocatively asserts that it on the contrary blatantly reveals that our society structurally relies on the incessant production of differential vulnerability and social inequalities.

To refer back to the 'interior' dimension of conformity and obedience vis-à-vis biopolitics, the pandemic period has also made a rather new theoretical contribution to the already burgeoning literature. The emerging concepts of 'democratic biopolitics' and 'populist biopolitics' can be mentioned in this context. The theoretical architects of both concepts pay obeisance to Foucault's formulation of biopolitics but go beyond it to catch up with the times – in a way making up for the guru's absence in the COVID-19 era. Toying with the idea of democratic biopolitics (and even in a step further, communist biopolitics) Sotiris (2020) suggests a 'different return' to Foucault in the current conjuncture by highlighting the role of social movements and collective decision-making – as foundations of the biopolitics from below. His point of departure is the now-familiar argument that the liberal democracies are unable to take stringent measures to counter the pandemic because they lack the same capacity for coercion or invest more on voluntary individual behaviour change. He is not convinced by this argument because he thinks that it is a simplification to pose the dilemma as one between authoritarian biopolitics and a liberal reliance on persons making rational individual choices. For him, protocols like quarantine or social distancing should not be treated simplistically as biopolitics because this kind of approach underestimates their usefulness as measures of public health particularly beneficial for the vulnerable groups. Then he moves on to present a utopian scenario in which the phenomenon of permanent individualised fear, a threat to social cohesion, is substituted by the 'idea of collective effort, coordination and solidarity within a common struggle' equally important to medical interventions in times of medical emergencies. It is definitely an ideal situation worth its place in the philosophical imagination. However, in the absence of any reference to the dynamics of the neoliberal political economy of knowledge and its co-optation mechanisms Sotiris perhaps becomes excessively optimistic, especially in visualising the democratisation of knowledge based on increased access and collective decision-making process – autonomous from the authority of experts. This warrants some discussion on my part on the neoliberal foundation of biopolitics and governance of our times.

In conceptualising 'populist biopolitics' Kirsten Schubert (2020) distinguishes it from 'traditional biopolitics' and therefore induces attention in this discussion. She claims that the traditional biopolitics in its focus on the repressive state fails to account for a new form of biopolitical normalisation that occurs during the pandemic: populist biopolitics, in her scheme, is a degenerated form of democratic biopolitics. According to her, it is bound to be so because populism marks degeneration of democracy. She further elaborates that it is a repressive and paternalistic form of democratic biopolitics, and it raises its head when the members of the community, and not the state, engage in biopolitics that limits freedom and normalises others. The most interesting and challenging part of populist biopolitics is that the members of the community indulge in mutual shaming – both online and offline – for supposedly irrational and unsolidaristic behaviour related to the disobedience of restrictive rules and norms like social distancing, stay at home and so forth. As if it is not enough, populist biopolitics, Schubert adds, also occurs in more formal political discourse, in such cases when the state itself is pressured to enact stricter regulations on the population. She identifies Germany as the prototype of populist politics and argues that low state repression facilitates demands for authoritarian measures. Regarding Sotiris' approach Schubert has a mixed feeling. She points out that while the 'young concept' of democratic politics has lot of analytic and normative values in being emancipatory, agentic, activist, pluralistic and participatory, and has the potential to reach biopolitical theory a lesson or two in these pandemic times the fact remains that it can go wrong and degenerate into populist biopolitics. What is of immense importance in the spirit and context of the discussion here is Schubert's admission that populist biopolitics in the epidemic times, in making moral and political calls in the name of the people – to do the morally right thing, to protect people by only resorting to the 'draconian social distancing measures' – exposes itself to the possibility of being misused by populist political leaders to establish authoritarian measures. She refers to the leadership in Hungary and Israel to illustrate her point.

Insofar as India is concerned, in the same issue of the publication in which Schubert writes, an Indian journalist (Ghosal, 2020:53–55) expresses apprehension that the central government in India might use the mobile app, *Aarogya Setu* (Cure bridge), launched in April, 2020, and operate on Bluetooth connectivity and access to the GPS data of the users to track COVID-19 infections. He finds it an 'easy tool' to track contacts and movements as the 'new normal'. The app has been linked by the Ministry of Home Affairs of the government of India to the public and private sector employees to gain access to workplaces and in some cases to get paid. It is also being used to get permission to fly inside India. The heads of the respective public and private organisations have been made '100% responsible' for ensuring compliance to the app. Though the central government, after coming under criticism from various quarters, decided to dilute the 'mandatory' clause doubts prevail about its intention. The report is based on the interviews of several activists and cyber experts, who agree that in the absence of any data security laws to protect the interests of the citizens there remains a distinct possibility of it being used by the ruling establishment for controlling the conduct of the citizens in the name of maintaining public health. This is notwithstanding the claim of the government of India that there are solid data protection principles in place to undergird the app. What is no less disconcerting is that the report mentions that the use of the app is being accorded wide support in the corporate media, a trend which, going beyond a rather simplistic description of the process as a 'governmental ploy', by itself implies some kind of collaborative venture between the state and the market forces. It is worth noting that in October, 2020, the Ministry of Electronics and Information Technology of the Government of India, responding to a query by the Central Information Commission (CIC), a statutory body which oversees the implementation of the Right to Information in India, disclosed that it has no information about the origin of the app. This invited a censure from the CIC and the mystery lingers on amidst the claims of strengthening transparency through digitalisation. It intensifies the apprehension that both transparency and accountability are sacrificed in the zealous pursuit of harvesting personal data of citizens by the government. Rights activists in India are also much concerned (Chandran, 2020) with the National Digital Health Mission, launched in 2020. While it seeks to be a repository of digital health records of the Indians the activists argue that in the absence of any data protection law and independent data protection agency it will only intensify citizen vigilantism. However, the cases being cited here are only fragmental manifestations of a much broader design of the biopolitical overdrive of information manoeuvring of citizens.

Information and citizenship: prefixing the 'bio'

The preceding analysis makes it amply clear that the strategy of the biopolitical overdrive has an inextricable link with bioinformation. It is also clear that governmentality also nurtures such link quite meticulously. Briggs and Hallin (2007:43–66), who seek to theorise (bio)communicability in the backdrop of governmentality, point out that governmentality lends them the idea that discourses constitute subjects and produce effects of power and freedom, locating subjects within social hierarchies. In locating and analysing the communicative dynamics in governmentality they state (p. 45) that the purpose is to explore how effects of power emerge from everyday ideological constructions of how information is purportedly produced, circulated and received, how individuals and institutions participate in this process, and how statements are infused with authority and value. Such link lies at the base of understanding Foucault's governmentality, and no less in understanding Agamben's 'state of exception' and 'bare life'. The link of biopolitics, bioinformation and governmentality, which remains an under-researched theme even amidst the prolific and ever-dynamic research on biopolitics, has always been there but here too the pandemic situation has brought in an unprecedented opportunity to the ruling regimes to calibrate it to their advantage. I would even go to the extent of noting without taking it to an extreme point that the complex of biopolitics/biopower and bioinformation aims at developing biocitizenship, a newly emerging concept in the study of what Foucault famously described as the 'conduct of conduct'. Acknowledging that a separate study is required for the theme, which is beyond the purview of this volume, let me briefly present their complex equations.

The discussion above also makes it clear that the conduct of biopolitics is also a venture in communication. Controlling the body and mind of the populations is impossible without creation, circulation as well as the simultaneous neutralisation of messages, meant for those whose lives are to be regulated in certain specific ways – with some protocols created by few for many. That information and communication in processed form have a vital role in the instrumentalisation of life and objectification of personhood is evident from the functioning of the biopolitical drive. A crisis situation, especially an unprecedented and disastrous one as the

COVID-19 pandemic, is particularly 'helpful' for the practitioners of governance because the messages carrying concern and the promises of safety, security, welfare, health and so forth will be taken much more seriously in such turbulent in such turbulent times. The anxiety, trauma, panic, grief and suffering, the relentless data generation of death lend considerable credibility to such communication, even if the messages may be of highly questionable character in terms of legitimacy. The governancing pattern during the crisis has shown a marked tendency to utilise the emergency situation not only to enforce but to normalise certain exceptional measures. With a mix of persuasive techniques but with the firm foundation of unilateral imposition of protocols the advocates of 'good governance' have resisted any protest against such imposition with strongest determination. Thus, when opposed, what would initially be projected as appeal would instantly transform into inviolable instructions or directives. In the name of welfare, safety and security of the populations no critical deliberations or debates would be allowed. The governing regimes would at best hear and not listen; at worst they would exercise coercion to bend the disobedient and the less obedient. There is encouragement to the feedback process in this regard, but it only has to be congratulatory in nature and not critical. The congratulatory response, as the case in India, may go to the extent of lighting lamps, bursting crackers, playing music with utensils, which are outwardly meant to appreciate the dedication and commitment of the frontline workers fighting the pandemic. But beyond it there remain traces of applauding the restrictive measures of governments. An analysis (Ghosh, 2021:1–20) of COVID-19 governance has empirically shown how in India the 'usual democratic channels' were sought to be bypassed through various omissions and commissions, giving rise to dialectical relations between policy communication and accountability. When it concerns the biopolitical governance on terror it has been shown (Edkins, 2008:211–232) that a number of intense protests by the relatives and activists of victims follow in the aftermath of the terror incidents. But there is a significant difference when it comes to a situation like the pandemic. Due to its prolonged if not unending duration and its consistency in taking toll on people its magnitude is far greater and the impact is far intense than what even a huge terror strike like the 9/11 can do. Under such circumstances there is little scope for resistance and protest by the people. What is no less important, as already noted, that people themselves may be convinced that such measures are not only required but need to be enforced with greater rigour. The 'natural advantage' on the part of the rulers to embark on such regulating strategy is that there is reason for supporting the concern for saving the life of people by governments under such threatening times, especially with life and death hanging in balance. At the same time it might bury under the heap of appreciation the concern that the protocols can threaten liberty of the people even beyond the pandemic times. Therein lies the fascinatingly intricate and intriguing part of biopolitics and bioinformation, and most evidently of the idea of biocitizenship. However, in the same breath it should be mentioned that much more studies on popular reactions are needed in the Surveillance Studies in general because, as has been noted (Saulnier, 2017:286–302) the theoretical understandings of how and why surveilled subjects perceive and react to surveillance, especially in the context of communicating relational messages, are rare in the field.

Whether and when such trends will usher in an era of biocitizenship (also known as biological citizenship) is a matter of debate and one need not be too eager to confirm that it will be soon. It is especially so because it is still a kid-concept in the theory-town of biopolitics. Describing biocitizenship as a 'complex and generative concept that allows scholars to delve deeply into the intersections of bodies with issues of agency, politics and resistance in a variety of contexts' Happe et al. (2018:1) start off with quoting Nikolas Rose's definition of the concept as 'all those citizenship projects that have linked their conceptions of citizens to beliefs about the biological existence of human beings, as individuals, as men and women, as families and lineages, as communities, as populations and as species.' What is important to mention here is that the concept has a conflicting character, something which I have mentioned about the mode of bioinformation during the pandemic. On the one hand, when it concerns the welfare, safety and security, especially with regard to health, and by implication to life, it has a positive attribute with welcoming gestures on the part of those for whom it is purportedly meant. On the other hand, when it is read in the biopolitical and bioinformational lens its negative attributes, as part of the disciplinary mechanism with the possibility of severe curtailment of rights and liberties of people come to the fore. It is noteworthy that even within a few years of the theorisation of the concept, after a degree of positive portrayal about its welfarist motive, some critical strands are surfacing slowly but steadily. There are reasons to assume that such a critical turn is warranted by the experience of governance-in-practice. Happe et al. devote a section to 'Biocitizenship Critiqued' (pp. 6–10) and endorse the emergent critique that scholarship on biocitizenship often neglects issues of social location, such as race, class, gender and disability. In doing so, they argue, it tends to promote individual health as a way of ignoring larger social inequalities. They also mention the underlying elitism and individualism characterised by the way the concept is theoretically formulated, and also the way the biotech industry is fed with certain kind of information facilitating consumption of its goods and services – arguing that all this threaten to replace active, collective engagement to create a better society.

The concept of biocitizenship then again has to be situated in the broader framework of neoliberal citizenship. It is not the place to engage ourselves in a detailed discussion on the trajectory of the neoliberal citizenship with all its historical accounts but the crux of the matter is that it does provide a stiff challenge to its observers. There are studies (including Rose and Novas, 2004:439–463; Plows and Boddington, 2006:115–135) emphasising the need to scrutinise biocitizenship against other contemporary citizenship debates. The logic for such stance is that in having had its source in biotechnology, including genetic technology and related information and in being propelled by the tremendous impact of the biotechnological revolution the biocitizenship approach in technocratic-reductive aggression may drive out alternative views and goals. Briggs and Hallin (2007:43) introduce the critical concept of sanitary citizenship – composed of the ways the states read bodies and bodily practices and assess the biomedical knowledge of individuals and populations – which constitutes an increasingly important site for regulating and rationalising access to privileges of citizenship. The concept of bio-communicability, mentioned earlier, provides an important guideline in this context when it draws attention to the ways in which, according to them (p. 46), the 'constitution of social subjects is embedded in ideologies about the "flow" of information and of discourse, about who constitutes biomedical knowledge, who is authorised to evaluate it and to speak about it, and through what channels it is assumed to flow.'

In its linkage with biopolitics it also has quite a significant relationship with knowledge and its political dimensions as communicability. It is stated to be producing a sense of freedom for some subjects, the right to acquire any knowledge, and for others the feeling of exclusion, subordination and constraint – the sense that 'information' is not directed at or accessible to them.

The challenge of producing critical theories of biocitizenship is stiffer because it has a superbly powerful sponsor in the neoliberal project. To provide a glimpse of the roots of such challenge, Mitchell's essay (2016:118–129) appears to be useful. She explores the subjectivity and governance of neoliberal citizenship as part of her concern with the multiple ways that individuals and populations are being detained, deferred, demoted, excluded or rendered as surplus from the citizenship norms, rights and from the sense of cultural belonging. Though her prime focus is on the western democracies at least the way she considers citizenship provides a fitting backdrop in the context of the discussion here. She defines (p. 125) citizenship as 'something that is formative of new ways of being – as a process that helps to constitute subjects in specific contexts.' While she goes on to examine the development and expression of neoliberal citizenship in the context of changes in the workings of capitalism, transformations in nation-state relations and shifts in forms of governing, all being our major reference points, she acknowledges the contribution of T. H. Marshall's classic study of social citizenship in *Citizenship and Social Class* (Marshall and Bottomore, 1992:8–17). However, she goes far beyond in the face of more complicated and even myriad patterns of the neoliberal variety. She views citizenship as a formation, which is constantly evolving and always constituted in relation to spatial and temporal processes and effects. To quote her (p. 127):

> 'While Marshall imagined a progressive future of increasing openness and inclusion, the actual workings of neoliberal citizenship indicate more complicated patterns. For some populations contemporary citizenship norms and practices have reflected and, in some cases, deepened forms of inequity and exclusion.'

It can be added that Marshall had set the ball rolling in having social citizenship as his locus, but he did not live long enough to witness how the millennial subjectivities, rationalities and technologies vis-à-vis the neoliberal governance would make inroads into the health terrain and how biopolitcs, bioinformation and citizenship would combine to mediate the body of the populations. To repeat, the process assumes extreme proportions when the populations show eagerness to conform to the restrictive measures. A study (Kloet, Lin and Chow, 2020:1–6) of the obliging tendency in South-East Asia during the COVID-19 pandemic, in Hong Kong and Taiwan, and also in mainland China, starkly reveals how a ready acceptance of the governmental advice or command demanding compliance to the health protocols easily and steadily morphs into a reassuring and self-congratulatory tone of the populations, taking much pride in 'we are doing it well, we are actually doing it better, better than others'. It is based on the unstated but no less vigorous premise that 'the more we are being controlled, the more we are in control'. The study calls it biopolitical nationalism, yet another addition to the repository of emerging concepts in the study of biopolitics, and inserts an interesting point that the virus is 'not only infecting, but also affecting'. The scholars admit that they are in an exploratory stage with regard to the question as to how biopolitics can become a field of competition, of rivalry, of nationalistic or, perhaps more generally, localist power games, in which the geopolitical entities that control the 'best' are being celebrated and praised, and those that fail are looked down upon. The findings of the study are echoed by Byung-Chul Han (2020b), who describes this as 'Asian advantage' and relates the authoritarian cultural tradition to Confucianism. Significantly, he points out that critical awareness of the digital surveillance is 'practically non-existent' in the region, and that there is little talk of data protection even in the liberal states of the region, Japan and South Korea. In this kind of ambience he identifies China as the front-rank holder and presents a future scenario, which he contemplates to be a result of the Chinese State and the Internet service providers in these terms:

> The State…knows where I am, who I am with, what I do, what I look for, what I think about, what I eat, what I buy, where I go. It is possible that in the future the State will also control body temperature, weight, blood sugar level, etc: a digital biopolitics that accompanies the digital psychopolitics that actively controls people.

Neoliberalism: pandemically ours

At this point of the analysis an effort may be made to situate the neoliberal project of governance with greater depth in the pandemic times. As a backdrop it may be reiterated that the COVID-19 pandemic has provided a great challenge to the neoliberal strategisation of health but at the same time the challenge is being well utilised for strategising further control. Žižek (2020b:13–14) poses a disturbing point in this regard when he notes that from a critical standpoint it is difficult to decide which is a greater threat to humanity: the viral devastation of our lives or the loss of our individuality in 'Singularity'. The debate may go on, but the fact is that the neoliberal project has shown remarkable attachment to reorganising the health sector, both locally and globally, to facilitate the processes of privatisation, commercialisation and financialisation of public services, including medical care. Its promotion of governance around the world is associated, as mentioned, with the practical implementation of the Washington Consensus. It is not that the act of governancing cares much for enlisting wide public support for such process, which its promoters know can never be guaranteed in the face of the wide scale deprivation and sufferings around. But at the same time they know that it is always a better option to have some degree of legitimacy, if it can be somehow managed. The pandemic has in a way provided such an option to be followed. Severe crisis of such disastrous proportions restricts the space and scope for critical-rational thinking and for resistance and protest, the topmost priority in such times being bare survival. The biopolitical overdrive of governance has shown its capacity not only in physically containing people and socially distancing them but also with a fair degree of success in overwhelming human interactions with digital interface, particularly in containing articulation of critical opinions on the infiltration and surveillance of the neoliberal parameters in the health domain. Social distancing, it may be argued, has to a certain extent contributed to the ambition of the neoliberalism-capitalism to change the whole texture of society with atomised individuals. To what extent it will have its impact in the post-COVID world, if there is one such world at all, should be a concern of social psychologists and is beyond the purview of this discussion.

Before noting how governancing utilises the situation it may be useful to refer briefly to the critiques of the modus operandi of the neoliberal project in the pandemic times. In an interview during the pandemic Achilles Mbembe (2020), the proponent of necropolitics, in response to a question highlighting the Brazilian President's ill-famed insistence on the preservation of economy even at the cost of lives, brings in and elaborates the concept of necroliberalism:

> This is the logic of sacrifice that has always been at the heart of neoliberalism, and it should be called necroliberalism. This system has always functioned with a calculating apparatus, the idea being that some people are more valuable than others. Those of no value are expendable. The question is of what to do with those we have decided are worth nothing. This question, of course, always impacts the same races, the same social classes and the same genders.

In visualising the post-pandemic times Mbembe makes an even more radical statement: 'There is no guarantee that we'll be here forever. The fact that it's plausible that life will continue without us is the key theme of this century.'

Describing noliberalism as a 'plague' of the most dangerous kind, another critic, Giroux, sets the background of the critiques in the specific context of the pandemic:

> The current coronavirus pandemic is more than a medical crisis, it is also a political and ideological crisis. It is a crisis deeply rooted in years of neglect by neoliberal governments that denied the importance of public health and the public good while defunding the institutions that made them possible. At the same time, this crisis cannot be separated from the crisis of massive

> inequalities in wealth, income and power. Nor can it be separated from a crisis of democratic values, education and environmental destruction. With respect to the latter, the coronavirus pandemic is deeply interconnected with the politicisation of the natural order through its destructive assaults waged by neoliberal globalisation on the ecosystem.

Notably, the core argument in such critiques is that COVID-19 has further exposed the absurdity of neoliberalism and the more radical versions of the critiques would go to the extent of predicting its death-knell. One can notice a number of positions and various shades in the emerging critiques. Let me now refer to some instances to substantiate the point. Foster and Suwandi (2020) refer to the rise of 'catastrophe capitalism', a 'late-imperialist' development of 'never before' interlinkages of ecological, epidemiological and economic vulnerabilities. The development, according to them, deepens the process of exploitation of the Global South as the production zones by the Global North which primarily concentrates production, finance and accumulation since the late twentieth century. As just stated, the most radical position confidently announces the end of the neoliberal rule. It may be called 'The End of Neoliberalism' thesis. How it is concerned is elaborated by Prashad (2020) in this way:

> Neo-liberalism of the earlier period offered hope—however illusionary—through ideas such as entrepreneurism and aspiration for upward mobility, as well as through the construction of desire for commodities which could enhance one's personal standing in the world. These hopes, however, are now crushed. They have been ground underfoot by financial and employment crises. In their place we have a zombie-like situation: The death of the ideal hope on the one hand, and at the same time, on the other, the existence of a callous hope that is crafted around hatred; a toxic hatred drawn from the old lineages of conservatism and tradition, and which sharpens its toxicity against women, foreigners, minorities and against anyone seen as the undeserving outsider.

Such stance assumes a more graphical form in an analysis (Saad-Filho, 2020) which describes the pandemic economic situation as the 'sharpest and deepest economic contraction'. The phenomenon is attributed to the collapse of the long supply chains that were previously the only 'rational' way to organise production, re-emergence of the 'hard borders', drastic decline in trade, severely constrained international travel, and unemployment of tens of millions of workers and the loss of employees, customers, suppliers and credit lines in business enterprises. All these factors are taken to be the sign of the reversal of globalisation – the supposed motive force of neoliberalism, which dismantles the state capacity. Analysing the sad condition in many countries, especially the grand triad of neoliberal governance – USA, UK and Brazil in their failure to cope with the coronavirus outbreak (and even to provide essential safety kits) and making a pathetic show of the efficiency – the analysis calls for effecting a 'desperate fight' on the part of the Left to eliminate the neoliberal-capitalist venture forever and establish an alternative society. Posing the question whether the pandemic can 'vanquish' neoliberalism Fazi (2020) remains quite hopeful. The argument is that the crisis has revealed how the nation-states, far from being powerless vis-à-vis markets, 'can jettison pretty much every rule in the neoliberal book', and that 'there's nothing markets can do about it, except beg governments for help'. It also advances the argument that governments remain the 'only actors capable of taking control of the economy when push comes to shove'.

In a much similar way there is another stance (Naidoo, 2020), which is not as emphatic in announcing the termination of neoliberalism but nevertheless projects the same outcome for the better future of 'both individual and collective wellbeing'. It is significantly influenced by the 'socialism or barbarism' thesis of Žižek (2020a) and a host of other scholars in interpreting the pandemic and it seeks to expose the paradoxes of the neoliberal-capitalist logic. It tries to do so by drawing attention to the way the power of the state is being invoked with the proven failure of the role of the free market to deal with the public health issue in particular and the welfare of people in general during the crisis. It identifies and visualises the fostering of collective solidarity, again in the Žižekian line, and points out that the choice never lies in choosing between 'liberalism now or later' or 'just strong state now, liberalism later', as both the options are no good. The aspiration inscribed in such stance is that the strong state must retain its strength without any possibility of rollback when the crisis is over.

Another position, for instance, that of Lapavistas (2020) which I would describe as a mix of socialism with semi-radical and pragmatic fervour does find absurdities in the way the neoliberal project utilises public health emergency for intensifying impact, but it does not see in it the end of neoliberalism. Lapasvitas discusses how neoliberalism in tandem with capitalism[1] is 'locked in its on absurdities', being incapable of transforming itself and how it resorts to the 'ever-greater doses of the same, disastrous, palliatives' for its own survival. But in a pragmatic vein he argues that there is a need to wage a long and winding struggle against it and against the 'threatening state', with the clear implication that the neoliberal absurdities are not going to eliminate its influence any time soon. It is a matter of further debate whether the working class, at least the way he conceptualises it, is ready to lead the struggle from the vanguard position. However, the fact is that such a stance reveals, from the perspective of a critic, the resilience of the neoliberalism-capitalism combine, which periodically faces crisis situations but refuses to go away.

There are some reformist critiques as well, which call for internal adjustments in the capitalist fold for better governance, without forsaking the path itself. For Mazzucato (2020), one representative of this position, the pandemic has come up with an opportunity to do capitalism 'differently'. She finds the governments having the upper hand in such crisis the moment must be seized to scale up governmental activities. She critiques the business-steered mode of governance and blames it for forcing governments to suffer from confidence-deficit and under-preparedness to face such crisis situations. Calling for the replacement of profit motive with public interest in governing she charts out a five-point stakeholder approach for better governance. First, governments must invest in, and in some cases create, institutions that help to prevent crises, and make us more capable of handling them when they arise. Second, governments need to better-coordinate research and development activities, steering them towards public health goals. Third, governments need to structure public-private partnerships to make sure both citizens and the economy benefit. Fourth, it is time to finally learn the hard lessons of the 2008 global financial crisis as various companies would come asking for bailouts and other types of assistance. She notes that it is important to resist simply handing out money and attach conditions to make sure that bailouts are structured in ways that transform the concerned sectors and they become part of a new economy and environmental protection.

There is yet another position, of a different genre from the aforementioned critiques. It is a temporary and tactical critique of neoliberalism by a proclaimed 'conservative neoliberal' assertion. Here, the basic argument (Reed, 2020), based on a time-specific detachment from the minimalist state, is that the debate over the Left and the Right have been made unnecessary by the pandemic. Distancing itself from any ideological contestation for the time being it advocates a stronger presence and role of the state, to recover from the hard-hitting unforeseen disaster. Though it does not equate this with 'setting capitalism aside and shunting to the left', and does not even float an admission that market economics has failed, such a tactical move towards greater governmental intervention is convened to move on. The interesting if not ironic twist in this critique is the expectation that the state needs to come forward, with support of the very rulers who made it slimmer on the grounds of 'minimum government, maximum governance', to resuscitate governance and protect its long-term interest of survival and sustenance.

There is little doubt that the manifold critiques of the neoliberal-capitalist mode of governing, filled with positive speculation and optimism, are needed to come out of the hopeless thought that nothing is going to change. But that does not solve the problem. The irony one finds in such critiques, all of which advocate in various degrees the 'return' of the state in a more proactive form, is their inadequate attention to two inescapable points: first, that the state in such times of neoliberal dominance cannot be the sole actor and it cannot but be guided by the advocates and activists of the market forces. Second, under such circumstances even if the state comes out of its slimming process and acquires a more vigorous interventionist role in determining the fate of people the way the pandemic has facilitated the scope for its biopolitical overdrive there is little possibility of the state playing the role of good old Samaritan – a role that is expected from it by the critiques. Lapavistas (2020) makes a candid observation on the complicit role of the state and its continuing importance in the neoliberal project:

> For one thing, the nation-state has always been at the heart of neoliberal capitalism, guaranteeing the class rule of the dominant corporate and financial bloc through selective interventions at critical moments. Moreover, these interventions were accompanied by strongly authoritarian measures, shutting

> people inside their homes en masse and locking down enormous metropoles. The state has also demonstrated its vast power to police society by collecting information through big data.
>
> This authoritarianism is fully in line with the dominant neoliberal ideology of the last four decades. State fiat is combined with the fragmentation of society as people are shut in their own homes and huge stress is placed on the individual responsibility to maintain social distancing. At the same time, large numbers of people are still required to go to work using public transport, while working rights are demolished, not least as layoffs rocket without concern for due process and as remote working destroys all limits to the working week.

Even after providing important instances of such state functions Lapavitsas admits to having remained 'unclear' as to what direction the global capitalism will take as it reels under the shock of coronavirus. He does see the possibility that colossal power of the state and its ability to intervene in both economy and society possibly resultingin a more authoritarian form of controlled capitalism in which the interests of the corporate and financial elite would be paramount. Importantly, he makes a call to the socialists to 'assess carefully and critically' the actions taken by the states to deal with the coronavirus crisis. Resonating him another critical observer (Achcar, 2020) of neoliberalism issues 'don't bet on it' advice on the question of self-extinction of neoliberalism.

All said and done, the pandemic crisis is not to be the treated as the end of the search for alternatives. As Lent (2020) points out, a crisis is a terrible thing to waste, and this crisis is to be manoeuvred for creating an alternative world order based on a 'transformed society', marked by meaningful participation of each one of us. He makes a plea to understand coronavirus as a political crucible, melting down and reshaping many of our current norms. Points taken, but the break between good intentions and practical implementation is found too often. Lent persuades others to 'think bigger' but he himself asks – what's next? – a difficult question without which the search for alternatives is meaningless. There are of course good intentions in the socialist critiques' call for a transformative state which is supposed to be driven by collective responsibility, solidarity, community engagement, community action and so forth. But exactly how it would come into being is not very clear. Apart from the fact that the fall of the neoliberal-capitalist states in near future is a distant possibility for many other reasons, no less because of the fact that even the officially socialist states like China, Vietnam and Cuba are being far more hospitable to the market forces than they were in the past. This trend considerably weakens the status of socialism as the gold standard in alternative governing. The above-mentioned excerpt from Prashad exemplifies the problem. There is much truth in what he writes about the pitfalls and failures of neoliberalism but when it comes to what he calls the 'validation of the socialist cause' by eliminating neoliberal tenets and practices from the face of the earth it entails an uphill struggle for the socialists. The clarion call for celebrating the death of neoliberalism-capitalism combine during the financial crisis in 2007–2008 has proved to be unfounded as neoliberalism continues to survive. Its capacity for mutation ensures its survival in more than one way. Referring to the excessive optimism about the impending downfall of the neoliberal project following the financial crash of 2007–2008 Mirowski (2013:1) presents a very realistic account in a slightly self-critical tone of the disappointing outcome in *Never Let a Serious Crisis Go to Waste: How Neoliberalism Survived the Financial Meltdown*:

> Fast forward to 2011. Whether it was true or not, people had just begun to hope that things were finally turning around. Moreover, journalists in mainstream publications bandied about the notion that academic economics had failed, and hinted that our best minds were poised to rethink the doctrines that had led the world astray. Yet, as the year grew to a close, *it slowly dawned upon most of us that the natural presumption that we were capable of rousting ourselves from the gasping nightmare, that we might proceed to learn from the mistakes and fallacies of the era of Neoliberal Follies, was itself just one more insidious hallucination.* A dark slumber cloaked the land. *Not only had the sense of crisis passed without any serious attempts to rectify the flaws that had nearly caused the economy to grind to a halt, but unaccountably, the political right had emerged from the tumult stronger, unapologetic and even less restrained in its rapacity and credulity than prior to the crash* (emphasis added).

Time and time again, the joint venture of neoliberalism–capitalism seems to have shown that the more they are cursed by the adversaries the longer they live. In the mid-19th century, Marx and Engels in *The Communist Manifesto* had asserted that capitalism digs its own grave. It seems that the grave is ready but still empty. This brings me to the point that amidst the surfeit of publications denouncing neoliberalism and capitalism, one finds lesser analyses of their survival strategy – how they face the periodic crises and still continue to survive. There are, however, some exceptional academic ventures though, such as, the wryly titled *The Strange Non-Death of Neoliberalism* (Crouch, 2011). Crouch's intent is candid enough when he declares in the Preface of the book that it is directed at those who have to cope with the world rather than those who try radically to reshape it. To encapsulate his approach, he does not resort to the familiar and widely used conspiracy theories in critically dissecting the trajectory and functions of neoliberalism. Crouch's approach is delicately poised because without expressing any pathological hatred for big corporations, which he sees as a 'third force' besides the state and the market, he shows, at some risk of being reductive in analysis, how they slowly but steadily infiltrate the state-market connection, and how with their 'business logic' they tend to influence the politics of both the Right and the Left.

To Crouch, the main actors occupying the world stage with their supranational jurisdiction are the giant firms. He defines (p. 49) giant firm as the 'one that is sufficiently dominant within its markets to be able to influence the terms of those markets by its own actions, using its organisational capacity to develop market-dominating strategies.' In another significant observation, of much value in the context of the fundamental parameters of the discussion in this book, he finds the manipulation of information and knowledge by giant firms, determining the contours of modern corporate behaviour in our times. This, he argues, in turn contributes to a growing asymmetry in government-people relations and to weakening the democratic norms – the public life as an arena for expressing and realising values – in governing. No less important, he adds (p. 56) that it erodes the democratic concept of 'consumer choice' with the technocratic concept of 'consumer welfare'. The 'citizens/customers' under the neoliberal regimes are deliberately left in the lurch insofar as information and knowledge are concerned. How the tech giants do it will be analysed in Chapter 5. On medical research Crouch's argument (p. 167) is that it can only prove its worth when a corporation succeeds in turning its work into clearly effective cures or into medicines that can be traded commercially. The latter observation is also relevant in COVID-19 pandemic times as one finds the unavoidable presence of giant corporations seeking to determine the fate and credibility of vaccines in their own terms. For Crouch, however, such trend is not surprising, considering the fact that the neoliberal political project has achieved much success in the corporatisation of 'more or less all' institutions like universities, hospitals, charities as well as governments, which have been put under an obligation to behave as though they were business corporations. On the 'astonishing departure' of neoliberalism, as distinct from liberalism, in its propensity to seeking close relationship with the state, he issues a warning note of sort. He argues (p.95) that the firms deliberately seek to forge such relationship as part of the strategy to influence the state to grant them favours and thereby serve their interests, rather than the other way round. In identifying the corporations as the core force in resilient neoliberalism Crouch frankly states that he holds no promise of a new social order – one which is different from the corporate-dominated one we are having – as an alternative. However, in what seems to be a compensatory gesture he visualises an 'open and vigilant society which might make life better' though it is not easy to imagine how it will materialise, especially after the way he illustrates the entanglement of state, market and civil society with the co-opting process of corporatisation and the leverage and power enjoyed by the giant firms.

In a later book, Crouch (2016) has his main focus on the 'knowledge problem' – highly distorted use of knowledge by corporations – something he discusses intermittently in the earlier book. In this case his argument is that neoliberalism is an 'enemy of knowledge' but it ensures its operation and survival through distortions of knowledge, with the avowed purpose of introducing the market-sourced malpractices to take over public service and public life. Though he claims that the market is not the sole source of dishonesty Crouch goes on to show how the knowledge distortion strategy, often led by the 'superior' projection of professional knowledge of the organised body of experts, and the 'market incentive to dishonesty', managed to come out of the financial crisis by manipulating knowledge. He puts forth (pp.2–3) five central claims as the base of this key argument. First, the attempt to make public services behave as though they exist in markets, a fundamental neoliberal policy achievement, leads to two results. It brings to those services an oversimplification of the knowledge involved in them and it also undermines the professions that are the carriers of that knowledge. Second, although the market is itself a highly elaborate form of knowledge heavy reliance on it undermines other forms, including the scientific knowledge that underpins much of modern life. Third, while early theories of the free market saw it as nested among actors who would act with moral integrity the contemporary form of market theory as rational choice exalts and rewards dishonest behaviour that connives at the corruption of knowledge. Fourth, while pure market theory requires an economy with large numbers of producers and consumers the actually existing neoliberalism accepts high levels of concentration of monopoly power, the domination of sectors of the economy by very few large corporations. In certain cases this also leads to powerful economic elites controlling access and distorting knowledge to serve their own interests. Crouch calls it 'corporate neoliberalism'. Lastly, the final distortion identified by him concerns the knowledge we have of ourselves. To act fully effectively in the market involves the process of being a 'self-centred, amoral calculating machine'. But there is a catch. As long as it is just one among a mass of features of ourselves it is not problematic. However, as the market and its analogues spread into ever further areas of life, we have incentives to suppress other features and to know ourselves primarily as these machines.

One does not have any doubt that the coronavirus pandemic has more than ever before exposed the market's inability to be self-correcting, contrary to what the neoliberal enthusiasts proclaim in the highest pitch. But the counter-strategy of bringing in a shadow nanny state cannot be taken at its face value as it results in an excessively optimistic view of the state as an entity bent on materialising citizen welfare. Here what Mirowski terms as the hard lessons of the financial meltdown of 2007–2008 may be relevant. Mirowski (2013:2) critically reflects on the misreading of the power of neoliberalism with these words:

> In 2010, we were ushered into a grim era of confusion and perplexity on the left. It took a rare degree of self-confidence or fortitude not to gasp dumbfounded at the roaring resurgence of the right so soon after the most dramatic catastrophic global economic collapse after the Great Depression of the 1930s. "Incongruity" seems too polite a term to describe the unfolding of events; "contradiction" seems too outmoded.

Thus, the enthusiasm that is generated by some scattered instances of the re-nationalisation of the health sector (as in South Korea and Ireland) or the re-nationalisation of AlItalia as the glowing evidence of the solid return of the state may miss the vital point that the neoliberalism-capitalism joint venture has a fairly long history of adopting an apparently one step back-strategy to eventually take several steps aggressively forward. To sum up, the turn-around of the neoliberalism-capitalism project – from the earlier perception of the state as a thoroughly incompetent and anachronistic institution to its change-over as a partner-in-need – has a much deeper motive reinforcing the survival instinct of the project itself.

Concluding remarks

What we thus see is that with the ICTs being hypothecated to the imperatives of governance the biopolitical overdrive has become an essential feature of the 'efficient' performativity of governance – engulfing social action – with unstinted support from the neoliberal project. Databanks are developed and promoted as perfect nests for collecting and preserving genetic informational codes, including the neural features and crucial psychological attributes, to serve the interests of informational capitalism, the cutting-edge form of capitalism in the global era. In a reductive and technocratic view of bodies as carriers of information the process facilitates the classification of populations for 'efficient' surveillance of their thinking and acting, and transforming life and the living substance of populations into objective economic categories. Behind the veil of such technologically sophisticated strategy lies the raw and crude motive of controlling and regulating the conduct of the population at will. The biopolitical trigger securitises individuals by injecting insecurity. The dismantling of public health, as exposed during and after the pandemic, reveals how the 'maximum governance' diktat minimises the life and liberty of people with permutations and combinations of homogenisation, differentiation and spatialisation at the micro-physical level. It is a typical manifestation of the 'offence is the best defence' strategy of the beleaguered campaigners and promoters of governance in the post-COVID-19 era.

Note

1 In this discussion and also throughout the volume capitalism is regarded as the economic organisation of neoliberalism. Lest such contention be misunderstood as an effort to put capitalism in a secondary position, it is also acknowledged that given the change in the objective conditions since the latter part of the 20th century capitalism in its own interest, in averting its crisis and ensuring its own survival, has reorganised itself and its inextricable accumulation process while adopting neoliberalism as its philosophical hub.

4

COMMUNITY, CRISIS, RISK

Communicating (dis)engagement

Introduction

The COVID-19 pandemic, as the preceding chapters reveal, is a much-complicated phenomenon in all possible respects. It is multidimensional, multilayered and, most of all, marked by many grey zones, which make even its best analyses inadequate. The knowledge about the outbreak and of the crisis it entails is at best partial. No one can afford to claim to have known the whole story even if on occasions there are efforts to maximise the role of experts and specialists to an 'uncontestable' extent in epidemic governance. The occurrence of the pandemic has coincided with the argument that along with the state and the market the community needs to assert itself and contribute to responsibility and care. 'Community consciousness', it is argued, should be a guiding spirit. The argument has its rationale in the sense that we need pandemic solidarity, and community is the best available means for it. But the issue at the ground level is much more complex. There is no doubt that 'community'[1] as a locus of supposedly shared interest and environment has a central place insofar as the crisis is concerned. The existing communities, whatever they are in whichever locations, tend to develop new 'cultural' orientations and behavioural patterns. The fear of having a diseased and infected body and the possibility of death of one's own and of others lend special depth to government-people relations. They are subject to greater control mechanism in the form of added regulations and norms to cope with the crisis situation – often as part of the promotion of the 'new normal'. There are also a number of mechanisms at work for cognitive co-option of community by the political establishment, some of which have already been extensively discussed. The pandemic's relations with the affected communities, with highly sensitive health issues at the forefront, add further angularities to the existing complications that mark the act of governing. It has been historically seen that whenever there is a crisis, imminent or actual, an intimate connection with

DOI: 10.4324/9781003247388-5

concerned communities is propagated by the policymakers, mainly in the form of a great concern for the wellbeing of people. It involves soliciting 'trust' to unleash a range of strategic measures to reorient behaviour of people on the ground that such times demand more than the standard administrative measures. Information becomes the most important tool in behavioural change in individuals and communities. The public runs the chance of being passive receivers in this process because they often lack knowledge of technical details of the crises and the associated risks. While it is true of crisis situations of all kinds, from war to natural calamities, it is especially true of health crises of such proportions such as the one under scrutiny here. In the case of health crisis the added dimension is the 'therapeutic' communication, in the broader sense of 'treating' people supposedly lacking information, the 'medicine' being the information flow sourced from 'the ones who know'. People are to be involved in compliance with minimal inputs from them, and they are not expected to be part of the 'top-notch' technical decision-making process. The known–unknown dialectics thus would take quite a complex turn insofar as this process is concerned.

It may not just be a coincidence that the literature on 'community engagement' has surfaced and intensified in the 1990s, when the same happened with regard to the governance paradigm. In course of time it has almost become a ritual to refer to community-engaged solutions in deliberations on crisis management and the theme has attracted attention of theoreticians and practitioners alike to a considerable extent in very recent times. Community engagement activities are sought to be integrated with the componential tasks of crisis communication and risk communication vis-à-vis the disease outbreak responses, all of which have also become an integral part of the governance discourse in general and health governance in particular. In this chapter, an effort is being made to situate and scrutinise such developments in the specific context of the coronavirus pandemic. In considering the engagement–disengagement paradox, with the vital issue of reconciling and/or negotiating 'engagement' with 'distancing', the ensuing discussion hypothesises that it may be more fruitful to view the paradox in the lens of communicative dynamics in crisis situations. This hypothesis may be related to a point mentioned in Chapter 3, that social distancing by promoting individualisation, to some extent serves the interest of the neoliberalism–capitalism project by weakening the collective fabric of society.

'Community' and 'engagement': the slippery slope

The concept of community engagement is different from what has traditionally been regarded as 'community mobilisation'. The latter is a necessary condition for the former which is supposed to have greater depth. In broad terms, community development is as an active, multi-way, dialogic and long-term relationship in which one party motivates another to get involved or take action – and both sides experience change. The major actors are the governments and the concerned communities, but there are also the allied stakeholders like political parties, NGOs, CBOs, philanthropic organisations, media, religious networks and so forth. In its idealised frame community engagement sounds positive and desirable, and this has significant implications for the known–unknown dialectics. Yet there are quite a few riders associated with it. First, there are power relations at play in determining the strength of the respective parties. Even if some kind of 'balance' would be ideal it is hardly found in reality, especially with the unavoidable presence of vast number of powerless people. There is no prize for guessing which among the two major parties – government and community–would be the dominant force in the community engagement process. Second, it may so happen that an ally, for instance the NGOs, becomes exceptionally strong and gets an upper hand in dominating communities to the extent of 'speaking for them'. Therein lies the role of what has earlier been described as the therapeutic approach. Which among the allied forces would take the upper hand cannot be easily predicted and much depends on the specific nature of the cases concerned. There may also be the lack of clear knowledge of the complex intersections of public interest, commercial interest, private interest and altruistic interest, and a strong possibility that such interests may mutate themselves with the passing of time. Third, there is no guarantee that communities are necessarily interested in engaging themselves in the process. Nor is there any magic wand to do so. Fourth, and most importantly for the discussion here, in the case of the devastating role played by such highly infectious and life-threatening pathogen like COVID-19 the demarcation between 'engagement' and 'disengagement' becomes confusingly blurred. The point can be explained in two ways. First, the very practice of community engagement in health crisis requires substantial degrees of physical disengagement in more ways than one. Thus, the regular physical connection that is considered so very essential for community engagement has to be dispensed with as physical distancing itself is part of the act of engagement in countering the health menace. Second, despite best of efforts to persuade and/or compel people to follow the regulatory acts and norms various instances of defiance are bound to remain. These two ways constitute the engagement–disengagement paradox. The paradox creates its own communicative dynamics through two related but contending modes – communication as a socially created and generated process, and as a techno-managerial means of 'social engineering'. A critical analysis of the complexities associated with community engagement praxis will be followed here by a critique of the crisis communication and risk communication to reveal how the pandemic exposes their deficiencies. Let it also be mentioned that the discussion would view the deficiencies in overwhelmingly political terms – to be gradually unfolded below.

Even to say that 'community' is a slippery notion is to make an understatement. 'Community engagement' is fated to remain a dicey process, particularly because it deals with human beings – to be more exact, human nature of perplexing varieties. How communities create and recreate themselves is a matter which has been a great concern of social thinkers of varying dispositions for a long time. The complexities at times threaten to shake the foundation of the concept of community itself. In what can be described as a highly radical interpretation of the community-centred communicative dynamics in the neoliberal era Byung-Chul Han (2020a) asserts that in the twenty first century the unobstructed march of neoliberalism gives birth to 'community without communication'. Han traces its guiding force in the free play of 'neoliberal psycho-politics', having its field among atomised individuals in atomised societies, in which collective feeling becomes a thing of the past. In his analysis community does not disappear in a literal sense but is subject to atrophy and commoditisation to such a scale that the symbolic elements that bind the members of a particular formation to develop and sustain community fade away. There are also other instances of substantially critical works with varying degrees of scrutiny of the notion of 'community'. Let me cite one such critique based a mix of philosophical and practical view of the concept of community, which interrogates the idealised version of the concept. In this critique, Iris Marion Young (1986:1–26), in advocating the construction of a radical political framework in understanding its collective dynamics, traces the problem in its idealised presumption that subjects can understand one another as they understand themselves. It, she argues, denies the difference between subjects. She comments (p. 2) that insofar as the ideal of community entails promoting a model of face-to-face relations as the best way it not only devalues and denies difference in the form of temporal and spatial distancing but also becomes undesirably utopian in several ways, one of them being the failure to address the political question of the relations among face-to-face communities. To quote her (p. 2):

> The ideal of community…totalizes and detemporalizes its conception of social life by setting up an opposition between authentic and inauthentic social relations. It also detemporalizes its understanding of social change by positing the desired society as the complete negation of existing society. It thus provides no understanding of the move from here to there that would be rooted in an understanding of the contradictions and possibilities of existing society.

It is evident that even the most radical interpretations are not yet making the 'end of the community' prophecies but are trying to persuade fellow analysts to discard utopian approaches, many of which ignore the vagaries of the contemporary times and take shelter in an idealised notion of community.

Generically, community engagement is an exceedingly complex idea as well as practice because it has a complex locus in 'community' itself. To accomplish the task, several requirements are identified (The Community Initiative Network, 2020) such as understanding and defining the social distancing context in which the communities to be engaged live, making certain any activities you undertake are safe for workers and communities alike, clearly defined objectives for engaging communities that listen and respond to community concerns as well as provide transparent and accurate information, focusing on vulnerable populations and the specific risks and challenges they face, and adapting, as much as possible existing networks, spaces for community engagement and approaches. The requirements are rooted in certain key factors regarding the compliance challenge. How people respond to these messages is driven by four key factors (Thompson, 2020):

i) Individual or group risk appetite. Risk appetite is how much of a risk one wants to take on a single or set of decisions or actions. The risk appetite of individuals to COVID-19 is driven by their knowledge of the impact and possible outcomes. Governmental risk appetite is driven with full awareness or knowledge of possible outcomes overlaid with political judgement as to what is acceptable socially. It is pointed out that at this point one begins to see the divergence of appetite: individuals and governments seek different outcomes, which involves limits to or loss of liberty versus saving lives and supporting public services. At one end of the spectrum there are individuals with a high-risk appetite, and at the other, governments managing the crisis and doing their best to mitigate all risks to spare healthcare systems and public services from being overwhelmed.
ii) Group (family or organisation) risk culture: in this, risk culture is more about awareness of the concept of risk at a social level. It takes account of judgement about 'acceptability', a struggle involving deciding and coming to terms with what is 'acceptable' in terms of possible outcomes. In the pandemic times it relates to a journey from low to high-risk culture in a very short space of time, which also entails a huge leap of mindset and change of thinking for many.
iii) Individual responsibility for consequential risk: this mindset change involves not only taking individual responsibility but also considering the consequential risk of the decisions made when it comes to assessing if undertaking a journey is necessary or can be worked out from home. In the context of COVID-19, it is added, this means the individual decision made can affect/infect many others. The complexity of this factor is recognised as achieving this mindset change is extremely challenging, especially when an individual's risk assessment focuses on own risk, rather than the consequential risk of being a potential 'super-spreader'. There are many instances of many remaining selfish and adopting a 'don't care' attitude about others.
iv) Counter-intuitive concept vis-à-vis the socially driven human race: the final challenge in communicating the social distancing message and drilling down compliance in a record timescale is to ask huge number of people to behave in a way that they are habituated with. It is counter-intuitive to the socially driven daily lives marked by physical contact through greetings, social gatherings, going to work and so forth.

The engagement process and its complexities can be viewed even more subjectively, under the lens of 'social character'. In a study the following characteristics delineated by Johnston (2018:22):

i) Cognitive engagement as an investment in attention, processing or thinking skills to develop understanding or knowledge. It among other things embodies the idea that humans can know or have knowledge either based on experience or based on reasoning.

ii) Affective engagement encompasses positive and negative emotional reactions such as enjoyment, fear, anger, support and belonging. It is often displayed as identification of belonging or emotional reactions. Positive or negative valence engagement reflects an inherent attraction or repulsion to an issue, leading to conditions for motivation, interest or concern.
iii) Behavioural engagement embodies the concepts of participation, collaboration, action and involvement. It also includes intended and unintended behaviours that may be caused by, or result from, cognitive or affective engagement. Scanning the literature one can assert that ideally community engagement has participatory impulse at its core, based on the premise that any official policy or authoritative decision can acquire greater scope for effective implementation and some degree of legitimacy with the involvement of people.

As noted by Reynolds and Sariola (2018:257), the suggestion in the literature on the theme, which has registered a surge in production since the last two decades, is that it has the potential to do a number of jobs: redressing past harms, dissolving long-standing mistrust and suspicion, minimising the risk of further exploitation, compensating for or resolve existing differences in power, privilege and positionality, allowing for marginalised voices and experiences to be represented in the production of scientific knowledge and ensuring relevant and impactful research.

One can further note that in such optimistic perspective the involvement of people can be engineered by way of providing their views and opinions, critical or congratulatory as the case may be, in the form of 'inputs', and the process can be maximised by people taking an active part in the decision-making process itself. Community engagement literature in its ideal form also celebrates the indispensability of 'shared knowledge', simulated by coproduction of knowledge among participants and 'shared learning environment'. It also claims to have laid primary emphasis on the upgradation of citizens from being silent onlookers to proactive participants. Relationships based on trust, inclusivity, transparency and responsiveness receive the highest priority in its agenda. There is also a belief, in some cases open and in some cases subtle, in the intrinsic 'goodness' of community and communication – a point which demands lot of qualifiers when put in the hard rock of reality. Community engagement involves action and action-related response. It is only obvious that communication holds the key to it. Community engagement and its communicative dynamics evidently encompass a mix of subjective elements and objective conditions. But the mix itself is problematic. As long as the perception and the reality-as-it-exists match they remain 'ideal' and the engagement process contributes to stability of some kind. But when a mismatch occurs, as it happened in the case of COVID-19 pandemic, the problem comes to the surface. The ideal stakeholder relations, the inter- and intra-community trust, trustworthiness of government and of various external agencies, systematic dialogue and so forth – all these issues valued by the mainstream community engagement communication literature – come under great strain. The multiple relationships in and among communities and those between the communities and the stakeholders become tenuous when an extraordinary crisis like the coronavirus pandemic strikes. The problem becomes no less complicated because crisis and risk elicit emotional responses of various kinds, with a range from compliance to defiance. Mis/trust in the motives and competence of the government come to play in myriad ways, with possibilities of swings, and the government on its part manoeuvres its 'authoritative' power to have an upper hand.

The designs of community engagement, along with an assemblage of methods, techniques and tools, aim at expanding the frequency and range of 'involvement' to elevate it to the higher stage of 'engagement'. It simultaneously boasts of several dynamic and open communication strategies, based on information sharing, which are devised and designated to deal with complex social, cultural and economic (and fleetingly mentioned 'political') environment. In order to show its open-ended character the community engagement literature acknowledges the complexities in having people at the centre stage of the process. To prove its proclivity towards democratic communication it highlights the importance of 'feedback loop' (which itself is a technocratic term, borrowed from the discipline of engineering). None would deny the vital role of collective agency in making decisions effective, but at the same time one also has to understand that creating and maintaining such agency in settings marked by a bewildering diversity is by no means an easy task. The tendency of a section of people to defy rules and norms has already been mentioned. Let me also mention here the issue of trust. There are societies, especially those characterised by scarcity, in which the trust level, both concerning people and government and concerning people themselves, tends to remain much below than what is required for efficient and effective management of the crisis. The problems acquire even greater complexity if one finds, as I shall now try to show, that there are some inherent constraints in the mainstream conceptual design of community engagement itself – something which was already there but has come to the fore with the outbreak of the coronavirus pandemic.

Community engagement: the 'action plan' spell

Even while underlining the importance of the steady emergence of the literature on community engagement I shall venture to make a critical observation that as far as its mainstream variety is concerned it bears an indelible imprint of 'action plan', marked by an obsession with preparatory positioning. In asserting this point I keep in mind the germination of 'other' instances of interpretivist and constructivist approaches in the literature. These approaches make efforts to address the existing and emerging challenges in the social setting and to transcend the dominant managerial traits in favour of ecological framework. They also seek to explain how democratic decision-making can be fostered by offering and utilising a conduit of voice, representation and collective-level influence. There is also a recognition (Johnston, 2018:19) of the perils arising out of the imposition of ideas and decisions on many by few and of the way they adversely affect the very goals of community engagement. In such studies communication tends to receive a special status, as a process which contributes to engagement by 'cocreating' meaning/s in outbreak times. The communicative foundation of community (re)orientation and the sociological roots of the contagion politics are reaffirmed in these studies (for instance, by Wald in Nixon and Servitje, 2016:vi) in this way:

> Communication shapes communities; the early sociologists at the turn of the twentieth century coined "social contagion" to express the material impact of the circulation of concepts and beliefs. Against the backdrop of the emerging field of bacteriology, microbes were both analogue and explanation for the emergence of social bonds: ideas and attitudes circulated like microbes, but also perhaps as microbes, as a not yet visible substance or energy. In all of its manifestations, contagion illuminates the connections that turn bodies into bodies politic.

But despite efforts like this the non-mainstream approaches and perspectives mainly remain confined to the theoretical deliberations and academic institutional sphere, with a rather limited impact on the ways community development is mainstreamed in a 'case book' like fashion in the policy precincts. This trend, however, raises some 'internal' critical queries about engagement communication about its viability.

One can in this context refer to a self-critical account by Heath, one of the pioneers in the field of community engagement. His essay (Heath, 2018:33–47) has an exploratory title 'How Fully Functioning Is Communication Engagement If Society Does Not Benefit?' Viewing engagement as the 'structure, function and discourse process' and emphasising its topical and contextual nature Heath issues the following warning (p. 39) against treating the theme too optimistically:

> Engagement is not some miraculous process. It is not an elixir to cure hostile relationships or a community's dysfunctional decision-making. It can lead to wise decisions that benefit all the members of a society, but it also can be enacted to serve a narrow interest, a "dark side" that may harm some for the benefit of others. It may be conspiracy against others' interests. Society's dysfunctions will frustrate engagement.

Here, one cannot fail to notice a similarity evident in having a 'wedge', as analysed in the previous chapter, between the conceptual-theoretical and practical manifestations of governance and in those of community engagement. When it comes to the community engagement in practice, which guides the actions in real-life situations the theme, as noted above, is subject to an action plan orientation. Several factors contribute to the process. First, as mentioned, it is based on a 'social engineering' approach, navigating the society towards attainment of some pre-set goals in gross managerial and technocratic terms. In such a scheme, society is in the background. Problems are posed and situated first, and thereafter solutions neatly carved out – mostly accompanied by liberal provisions of 'tips' and references to 'best practices'. There are indeed references to the problems, 'noise' in the case of communication flow, but they would invariably end with a set of 'viable solutions' based mostly on certain specific formulae. Second, and it is related to the first point, like case books with action plan orientation, the mainstream literature on community engagement is overwhelmingly made up of practice problems, mainly sourced from different contexts if not outrightly from the imaginary ones. Third, the way action plans compulsively repose trust in some 'authoritative' sources, in the visualisation of community engagement in the literature, even if communities are apparently persuaded to play a direct role, the ultimate leverage and agency are vested in the authoritative source of government. There are direct or implicit assumptions that communities are to be 'geared', a basic postulate of the social engineering thesis. Fourth, and by no means the least important, the community engagement literature, particularly those portions which dominate its operational form, either steers clear of political issues or at best provides a peripheral space to them in comparison to the social, cultural and economic factors and issues. The marginalisation of the political parameters and dimensions not only results in underestimation of local political dynamics vis-à-vis community engagement but also moves the focus away from the larger story of the state-market dynamics of the new millennium. Moreover, it runs the risk of confining the explorations of community engagement at surface level by avoiding deeper investigations of its purposes and modes, and even at times circumventing the foundational question of who are included and excluded in the orbit of 'community'. In brief, who sets the terms of such engagement and how remain ambiguous and beyond the entitlement of knowing. The dynamics and dimensions of community engagement, if interpreted apolitically, suit the action plan orientation and promise a rather smooth preparatory agenda as the 'disruptive' power relations coming in the way of fast implementation of governmental policies and decisions are evaded.

The most widely circulated definition of community engagement, made in the context of public health by the Centers for Disease Control and Prevention (CDC), the national public health institute of the US, substantially reveals the action plan orientation. In the definition (CDC, 1997:9), community engagement is defined as a process of 'working collaboratively with and through groups of people affiliated by geographic proximity, special interest or similar situations to address issues affecting the wellbeing of those people. It is a powerful vehicle for bringing about environmental and behavioural changes that will improve the health of the community and its members. It often involves partnerships and coalitions that help mobilize resources and influence systems, change relationships among partners, and serve as catalysts for changing policies, programs and practices.'

The definition also reflects a futuristic orientation basically revolving around the ways and means of improving the existing situation with reference to certain key elements – knowledge generation, skill formation and capacity building, coalition building and so forth. If this is the case, there is not much confusion about the fact that in the case of a sudden outbreak of a gigantic phenomenon like the coronavirus pandemic the preparatory process would be suspended as it would prove to be 'unworkable' in the wake of several new rules and norms as part of the 'new normal'.

Let me refer to five major steps of community engagement-in-practice to further reveal its action plan orientation. The steps are (DELWP, 2015:3):

i) Informing the community of policy directions of the government.
ii) Consulting the community as part of a process to develop government policy, or build community awareness and understanding.
iii) Involving the community through a range of mechanisms to ensure that issues and concerns are understood and considered as part of the decision-making process.
iv) Collaborating with the community by developing partnerships to formulate options and provide recommendations.
v) Empowering the community to make decisions and to implement and manage change.

There is little doubt that all the steps are important not only for enlisting the importance of community-sensitive engagement but also for sustaining it. At another level, they also reveal the importance of communication, though mainly as an instrumental force. But the moot question is how free and democratic the process is in terms of, for instance, the crucial issue of access to information. The question is important as it goes on to determine the degree of opportunities for participation. Viewed from a managerial angle there could be nothing more democratic than having the recognition of the aforementioned steps. However, a critical focus on the same, arising from an ability to read the fine print in such steps, will show that such conclusive note may be too simplistic. The action plan orientation in having an 'ultimate' authoritative source to manage things is strongly embedded in the fine print of the steps – in making the government, and not the community, the undisputed game-changer. It also runs the grave risk of circulating information and data considered 'relevant' and 'appropriate' by those who control the leverage of power. If the source, namely information and data, is manoeuvred all the stages mentioned here would be automatically manipulated with a smokescreen of engagement.

My motive here is not to undermine the importance of government, but to draw attention to the point that any uncritical reliance on it as the game-changer complicates much of the participatory impulse of community engagement initiatives, including its communicative dynamics. To be more precise, the aforementioned steps show that there are various ways in which information, and communication as its processed form, is necessary to achieve engagement in a 'shared environment' and it may be taken as a means to reach the final goal of empowerment. However, what remains largely hidden in the apparently impressive format is the point that with such superordinate status provided to government, by a broader implication with the state being regarded as a kind of benign behemoth dedicated to the welfare to people, the power relations become highly inequitable. Such inequitable power matrix constrains the possibility of the emergence and sustenance of new democratic spaces from the ground below and paralyses the radical potential of popular involvement and its elevation to the status of engagement. It also gives rise to the possibilities of community engagement being manoeuvred to serve narrow political interests of few, especially those managing the state/government (and not to forget the market forces). Even if there are many instances of community development literature referring to 'political environment', 'political factors', 'political coalitions', 'political norms' and 'political actions', interestingly no detailed discussion, required by the complexities of the issues concerned, is to be found. But it is only symptomatic of the larger scenario, of evading complexities beyond a 'manageable' point. Thus, in a critical essay meant to strengthen the case for community engagement by identifying some of its basic deficiencies, Dempsey (2010:360) notes that 'the existing discussions on the theme downplay the complexity of community, abstracting and dissolving important divisions and power structures in the process.' She adds that as a result, they misleadingly assume rarely existing unity and homogeneity. Though the essay has the specific context of the (university)campus-community divide the observations made in it have broader significance. Consider, for example, another observation by her (p. 365, emphasis added):

> The need for community perspectives on engagement is made even more problematic by the *uncritical way* in which the interdisciplinary literature conceives of community. Existing discussions of community engagement downplay the complex nature of community by treating it in the abstract. These abstract treatments are misleading in that they assume an amount of unity and homogeneity that rarely exists… Abstract treatments are particularly problematic when they result in essentializing conceptions of community.

Dempsey acknowledges the 'popularity' of community engagement but that does not deter her from pointing out (pp. 365–366) a 'significant drawback' of treating community in the abstract in the concerned literature. She argues that abstract calls for greater engagement with local communities prompt questions about the politics of voice, including who may speak on behalf of a particular community, and that such abstract treatments also imply that locating and representing a community's interests is non-problematic. On the other hand, a direct acknowledgement of the diversity of community opens up new understandings of the politics involved with identifying and representing community interests. In this way, critical perspectives on community introduce an important set of concerns about who (and what) constitute the community within the sphere of community engagement. She also alerts the mainstream academics about the detachment of theory and reality, as being reiterated here. Dempsey treads the path of knowledge dynamics vis-à-vis the universities as knowledge hubs by providing certain recommendations for more effective community engagement. She concludes with four sharp recommendations of significant implications for introspection on the theme. First, creating ethical modes of engagement and making blunt assessment, including the acknowledgement of the ways in which concentrations of wealth and power/knowledge already engage their surrounding communities. Second, enunciating active measures to surface issues of difference between and among participants to recognise and plan for the heterogeneity of community as well as the difficulties involved with identifying and representing a community's interests. This she suggests can be done by incorporating processes of dialogue and deliberation whereby members are able to recognise their different positions in relation to one another. Following this trail in communication she specifically refers to the need for scheduling time for reflexive communication about the terms of engagement, taking also into account the impact of economic, social and historical processes on their current relationships. Third, she mentions the need to adopt measures to anticipate and actively mitigate the ways in which community engagement efforts reproduce existing material inequalities within and between communities. Fourth, she notes that given the tension-filled nature of community change when it comes to community engagement efforts there lies a requirement in the form of willingness on the part of its participants to engage in the murky and contentious process of pursuing mutually transformative programmes for change and also as part of this endeavour, of 'revisiting' local politics.

This is what I am trying to note – that howsoever well-meaning the non-mainstream theoretical genre of community engagement is it cannot prove its analytic worth if there is a divorce between theory and practice, and unless the formulations are tested for effectiveness in real-life situations, especially in emergencies and more particularly in health emergencies. In the case of a severe crisis like the coronavirus pandemic the 'transformatory' promises of community engagement would witness formidable twists and turns, so much so that they will have little scope to justify their existence. The pandemic-related developments, however, are anything but one-sided. On the one hand they generate the scope to manoeuvre the engagement factor to the advantage of the dominant forces, especially of the ruling regimes. But on the other hand they also nurture various forms of destabilising communication flows to challenge the dominant mode and on occasions even to sabotage it. I prefer to call the latter variety 'subversive communication', which will be taken up for discussion in the next chapter. The vital point to take note of is that none of the two varieties contributes to the credibility of the prevailing theories of community engagement. Despite their conflicting ramifications both reveal the constraints and limitations of its conceptualisation. To refer to the dominant approach to community engagement once again, it does remain aware of the political environment as a 'barrier', but being overwhelmingly concerned with promoting an 'enabling environment' with some haste it only makes scattered and cosmetic references to the political complexities. There is hardly any attempt to take up the 'political' head-on to reveal its great potential in manipulating both 'community' and 'engagement' and in deviating community engagement from its idealistic, redemptive and emancipatory plane.

Making a case for community and communication interface and noting that communication plays a key role in shaping community since the ancient times Shepherd and Rothenbuhler (2013:ix) nevertheless highlight the 'stunning diversity' in the theoretical and empirical trends in the interface and the 'daunting' task of addressing it:

> Community is found in time or place, in networks or relationships. It is used to control; it is freeing. It is the basis for democracy itself, or a cover for repression. Although some see community entering a new age of access, growth and vitality, many others see it withering away.
>
> Communication, too, can be this, that and the other thing. Communication is conceived as the necessary symbolic base of community, and, in the form of mass-produced entertainment as the number one distraction from community. Communication can be understanding, empathy and relation; it can also be propaganda, ideology and manipulation. Communication can be the very model of democracy, or the very method of its subversion.

Considering both sides of the coin Shepherd and Rothenbuhler emphasise on understanding the importance of locality in a rider to comprehend the nature of communication. In doing so they focus on the importance of materiality. They argue (p. x) that the material bases of community are often overlooked by communication scholars and that they are easily taken for granted even if no community and no communal relation exist without an enduring material base which provides the situation in which, and the conditions and resources of which, communally directed communication is constructed and engaged. In a further move towards more nuanced and complicated relations between community and communication they refer (pp. xi–xii) to a set of pertinent questions: i) Should we assume either communication, community or both to be inherently good? ii) What is required for either or both to be experienced as good?

In raising these sensitive questions and putting them at the core of their analysis they also take shelter in John Dewey's proposed criteria in *Democracy and Education*, written in 1916, for judging the goodness of any community – first, how numerous and varied are the interests which are consciously shared? The second, how full and free is the interplay with other forms of association? What Dewey proposed seemed to have clear reverberations a century later, not because he has been heeded much but because the ethical and political mix of the questions has been left unaddressed to an extent, that too with many implications for the known/unknown dialectics. That such lag exists in a major way is evident when Reynolds and Sariola (2018:268) express in such words their concern while exploring the complex relational dynamics of ethics and politics in global health research:

> Despite explicit objectives related to socially responsible knowledge production, inclusivity, and empowerment, practices of community engagement in

> global health research are not inherently democratising… (C)ommunity engagement programmes can serve a wide variety of ends. Engagement activities can be used for purely instrumental goals – to gain community 'buy-in', to increase consent and study enrolment, or to ensure smooth research operations – rather than to achieve broader transformations in the politics and power dynamics of research. Further, despite the inclusive promises of community engagement, engagement practices can be exploitative or can serve to exclude already marginalised members of a community… Instead of redressing ethical concerns around research, engagement activities can introduce new ethical and social challenges [emphasis added].

One of the most important points mentioned by them, which assumes much greater proportions in the context of the COVID-19 pandemic, is that people involved in 'community engagement' activities might have nothing in common except for a shared disease diagnosis or increased risk of contracting a specific disease. In other instances, 'communities' may be constituted temporarily or fleetingly, as those who are brought together for a particular activity or engagement event. Incidentally, Reynolds and Sariola do not rule out the possibility of engagement being a 'window dressing' or masking unequal power relations facilitating the imposition of a form of governance or a particular political ideology.

At this juncture of the discussion the WHO's perspectives on (global) health governance, and particularly on community engagement, merit attention. The debate on the organisation's effectiveness goes on unabated also in terms of its approach to communication in COVID times. Even the WHO guidelines fall short of addressing the risk communication issues. Thus, one finds scholars (French and Monahan, 2017:4) arguing that the guidelines remain silent on how risk communication messages propagate through deeply surveillant media and social media networks, thereby resulting in an inadequate understanding of the surveillant dynamics during the COVID-19 times. There is a related plea (p. 5) for enhanced theoretical understanding of the ways the pandemic anxiety creates 'dis-ease' in several different registers. There are also more specific pleas: to consider how COVID-19 is reconfiguring cultural understandings of bodily vulnerability, social processes of stigmatisation and marginalisation, structural inequalities and forms of structural, everyday violence, which predispose people and communities to the harmful effects of communicable disease while also undercutting their capacity to respond to these effects; and also to consider the role played by public health and other authorities in disease construction as well as the problems, unintended consequences and issues arising out of their efforts to detect, pre-empt and contain disease spread. However, without undermining the criticisms of its modus operandi it may be mentioned that as such the task of finding some generic recommendations vis-à-vis the global health governance is, to say the least, challenging. Tracing the roots of the global health governance since the mid-nineteenth century Zacher and Keefe explain (2008:135) why it is so:

> Contemporary global health governance is complicated and messy; it is comprised of numerous and varied actors with competing values, interests and motivations. Even the goals of establishing a strong health governance regime are varied and contested. For some, the predominant goal of a strong health governance regime is to reduce the incidences of death by infectious diseases; for others it is to bring about improved economic development; for others it is to increase security against the threat of infectious diseases; and for yet others it is to develop a health policy that does not impede the flow of global trade and commerce. Depending on which goals or values the actors prefer, they will employ different control strategies.

As far as the WHO is concerned a scrutiny of what is regarded as its most important and comprehensive document on health governance, The World Health Report 2000 (WHO Report I, 2000), provides important cues on how the apex global organisation of public healthcare constructs its roadmap on health governance, and where it falls short in such endeavour. The report has as its central theme 'Health Systems: Improving Performance'. It refers (p. 13) to the historic Alma-Ata Declaration (1978) which had adopted primary healthcare as the foundation for achieving the goal of 'Health for All', and it promises to reinvigorate efforts to deliver basic healthcare to people everywhere. The report makes a critical observation on how the mainstream approach to the primary healthcare movement pays 'too little attention' to people's *demand* for healthcare and how it concentrates almost exclusively on their presumed *needs*. It also notes that the systems fails when the two concepts do not match, and the supply of services possibly fails to align with both. Such contents raise the hope that community engagement will be visualised as a possible solution. But significantly, the report has no reference to it – neither in this specific context nor throughout the text. A number of times 'community' has been mentioned in the report but mostly with the goal of advocating the case for 'community pooling' in healthcare system. I shall return to this point soon. Here, one may consider its time of publication, the new millennium, and the then emerging political economic contours. The report significantly argues (p. 15) that the inadequate attention to the demand factor is reflected 'in the complete omission of private finance and provision of care from the Alma-Ata Declaration, except insofar as community participation is construed to include small-scale private financing'. This contention confirms the point, which is set forth (p. xiv) at the beginning of the report, that health policy and strategies need to cover the private provision of services and private financing, which are to operate side by side state funding and activities. It calls for an end to the hitherto dichotomous relations between public financing and private financing and rationalises the collaboration of the two. There is a firm conviction that 'only in this way' can health systems as a whole be oriented towards achieving goals that are in the public interest. Interestingly, the report does so in the background of the observation that a health system in which individuals have to pay out of their own pockets for a substantial part of the cost of health services at the moment of seeking treatment clearly restricts access to only those who can afford it, and is likely to exclude the poorest members of society. But there is no blueprint as to how the reconciliation of the public and private financing would be made. The absence of such guide is pertinent to the discussion here because what we witness in the new millennium in particular is the reverse and invincible swing towards for-profit healthcare as part of the broader strategy of subjecting public interest to the market logic, and the consequent shrinkage of the state provision for healthcare. Needless to say, it has an immensely adverse impact on the life of ordinary people, especially the underprivileged sections of the society. How to implement in practice the lofty ideals of community engagement theories in such times, when the act of governancing marginalises the competing ways of seeing and knowing and the dissonant 'voice' of people at large, is a question still in search of an answer. The answer cannot not be found in the report as it treats the 'political' only cosmetically and does not explicitly relate health governance to the gross imbalance in social opportunities that pervades the eco-system of most states of the world and aggravated by the advent of market reforms.

That community engagement is a blind spot in the report is not surprising because the WHO in general has been rather slow in taking up the issue. After dallying with the concept for a while it began searching for a suitable framework of the same and the search intensified since the outbreak of the Ebola virus in the African states of Guinea, Liberia and Sierra Leone in 2014. A concrete community engagement framework – known in the WHO parlance as the CEQ (Commitment to Equity) framework – emerged in the organisation's report, titled 'WHO Community Engagement Framework for Quality, People-centred and Resilient Heath Services' (WHO Report II, 2017). Its rationale is explained thus (p. 25):

> The CEQ framework recognises that strength in any system comes from connections. This is especially the case with human systems. If healthcare systems are to exhibit strength and resilience when tested, they must be built on strong interconnections between healthcare professionals and community members. To create and sustain such a system, each must work together, sharing information, building trust, and engaging each other in such a way that the concerned goals become mutual, and everyone feels empowered to contribute to the system's success. To enable such connections, leadership needs to be imbued with a knowledge and vision of how such a system can be created, developed and constantly evolve as the needs of the community and the demands on the system change. More specifically, all members benefit from using an analytical framework that recognises the need for mutual engagement, empowerment and also realises that every circumstance is best managed in a context-specific manner. Further, each person is well served if they develop strong collaborative skills so as to be able to engage across communities and societies, to effectively move through

> conflicts, to craft policies, procedures and practices along with the necessary monitoring and evaluation, to achieve constant quality improvement in the system and in health indices. These analytical frames and engagement skills can be taught and improved throughout the system, from each and every professional to all community members. Widespread skill is truly the underpinning component of empowerment that in turn, enables the strongest and most resilient system.

One can see that even in this framework of community engagement the political component has retained its minimal position. The excerpt shows that the framework has provided much attention to the possible contribution of community engagement but how to navigate it through the political terrain remains unaddressed. One may argue that given its character, the WHO is not exactly an organisation which can afford to throw much light on the political factors. This may be true but the catch is that without having such scope its discourse on community engagement would at best remain a piece of 'theoretical' action plan.

The huge challenges faced by the advocates of community engagement communication are also the ones that confront crisis communication and risk communication, which are even more specially designed for the tumultuous and highly uncertain times caused by disasters and/or outbreaks. The following section highlights the predicament of that context. In this case too, as shall be shown, there is dominance of technocratic orientation, which comes in the way of the realisation of potential.

Crisis and risk communication: on overcoming the 'toolkit' bias

The two concepts 'crisis' and 'risk' are closely related as crisis is broadly defined as risk gravely manifested at a particular point in time. In the following discussion crisis communication and risk communication are linked with one of the most the complex and challenging tasks of governing – that of raising public awareness about the pandemic and controlling anxiety, fear and panic among people. There are obviously no instant techniques for countering this challenge.

There is no doubt that ideally communication during grave crises is expected to dispel ambiguities and confusions about what exactly the situation is and where exactly the risks lie. It demands converting a number of unknown elements into the known. But it does not seem to be the case with the COVID-19 pandemic. Consider once again the case of 'social distancing' which has played its role in enabling the pandemic to generate confusing signals from its outset. Within few days of the outbreak it achieved wide circulation to become part of the 'COVID lingo'. It has also been part of the advisories of most authoritative sources like the WHO, governments, NGOs and CBOs, generating wide publicity as the 'best defence' against the pandemic's cascading effects. Within few weeks the social distancing norm became the 'new normal' all over the world. Its defiance would invite punitive measures from authorities, apart from aggravating the risk of getting infected with the virus.

As a restrictive measure it in some instances resulted in agitations. On rare occasions, as in Sweden, the government, following only the epidemiological guidance, undermined its potential and decided not to pursue it except for the elderly. It did not, however, augur well for the country as it began facing a high mortality rate from late 2020, and was forced to introduce lockdown. The Canadian government gradually phased out the term 'social distancing' from public pronouncements to avoid confusion. There were cases of 'unmasked' people indulging in street protests and even of throwing 'coronavirus parties' against its imposition, on the ground that it violates fundamental rights and freedoms. Social distancing has also led to few write-ups critical of its nomenclature and of its ambiguous role. Let me refer to one such instance. The following excerpt from a letter written by two concerned scientists (Das Gupta and Wong, 2020:488–489, emphasis added) to governments and the media, with an appeal to replace the term with 'physical separation' not only deals in strong words with the problematic outcome of the concept but also refers to the communicative dimensions of the same:

> Nations around the world have been urging their citizens to practice "social distancing." It has become the moniker for what we "need" to do to fight the COVID-19 pandemic. However, *social distancing is a misnomer. It is not self-explanatory, conceptually ambiguous, practically misleading, and intellectually misplaced*... In public health, social distancing refers to community infection-control measures to achieve physical separation by restricting movements of and contacts between individuals during outbreaks... Thus, practices of social distancing are purely physical-spatial with nothing social in nature...
>
> Some have supported the continued use of social distancing because it is now a familiar phrase, and switching to a more physical term may no longer be needed... Any such claim founded solely on the current context is short-sighted. The succession of zoonotic pandemics in the twenty-first century directs us to a longer-term outlook for better public health preparedness. Moreover, *rapidly evolving global events require sharing of information across cultures and disciplines, but the misleading nature of the term inhibits this communication.*
>
> Removing social distancing from the public health vocabulary and replacing it with a term such as physical distancing or separation would ensure unambiguous health messaging and avoid further academic confusion.

It is evident that the problem with social distancing is not just a problem of nomenclature. It is a problem of much bigger proportions, involving the efficiency and effectiveness of policy communication in catastrophic times. In other words, it is only symptomatic of the deeply rooted issue of conducting crisis communication and risk communication. However, these counteractions could not prevent it from being part of our common sense of safety in everyday life during the pandemic. It can also be noted that on the technical front the debate on social distancing was mainly concerned with the technical measurement of the 'preferred distance' to maximise protection and not as such on its viability. What is of much significance both as a concept and as a norm social distancing inscribes a paradoxical essence – that in actual terms it means physical distancing. It does not require much brainstorming to get through the point that in the proper sense of disengagement from social interactions it is an impossible venture insofar as our existence is concerned. It is particularly so because as noted above the crisis times are invariably fused with calls for community engagement, formal or otherwise.

The main argument in this section is that in tackling the pandemic situation the fundamental condition of policy communication is that it has to move beyond the 'toolkit approach' and follow the dynamic and transactive path. The toolkit approach is basically a marketing technique, which provides one-size-fits-all kind of solutions to the problems, existing, emerging and speculated. It enjoys high status in the world of marketing and is widely used. However, the question is to what extent it can be superimposed on a society which is not only a much larger entity than a firm but also has an exceedingly complex mode of operation than what is found in the market arena. The act of governing along with policy formulation and policy execution is by any means a far larger and much more complex task than what are considered marketing activities. Even the best tools and models in the toolkit approach, developed originally with firms in mind, turn out to be too simplistic to negotiate the cobweb of society. Explaining how the close yet complicated linkage of risk, uncertainty and the unknown–unknowns of unstudied or unstudiable conditions give rise to a politics of uncertainty a study (Roe, 2020:73–84) makes conceptual distinctions between controlling, managing and coping as operational outcomes. Three types of unpredictability are identified (pp. 76–79):

i) Risk probability and consequences of failure are known and estimated.
ii) Uncertainty: either probability or consequences of failure are unknown or not estimated.
iii) Unknown–unknowns: neither probability nor consequences of failure are known for estimating.

The operational outcomes are:

i) Control: low and stable output variance through keeping low input variance and low process variance.
ii) Manage: high input variance matched by high process variance to ensure low and stable output variance.
iii) Cope: high and unstable output variance and/or inadequate process variance to match input variance.

The study reveals a greater and timely realisation among scholars that neither direct nor indirect variables of the politics of uncertainty need to be further qualified to negotiate the highly unsettling times.

It is true that social theory plays a part in understanding crisis communication, as it also does when it takes up uncertainty and risk as a theme. The much-needed initiation in this regard was provided by the unorthodox "Risk Society" thesis by sociologist Ulrich Beck[2] whose prime concern with environmental hazards (Chernobyl in particular) also led him to deal with the political dimension and positioning of knowledge vis-à-vis risk. To provide just one but a very important dimension of knowledge politics as discussed by Beck (1992:23,53), he vigorously analyses the differentiating roles of consciousness by observing that while in class and stratification positions it is the being which determines consciousness in the case of risk positions the case is just the reverse. He describes (pp. 23–24) this as 'new political significance of knowledge' and claims that accordingly the political potential of the risk society must be elaborated and analysed in a sociological theory of origin and diffusion of knowledge about risks. But with certain exceptions, as distinct from social theories of risk and uncertainty, Beck is either missing or at best has a marginal status insofar as the dominant mode of analyses in crisis communication and risk communication is concerned. There are two major reasons for this. First, he has much regard for the 'political' in his analysis in which he traces the roots and dimensions of changes from class conflict to risk conflict vis-à-vis discriminations and scarcity in society. Second, his unit of analysis is much broader than what it is in the case of the mainstream literature in crisis communication and risk communication. To reiterate, a distinctive feature of the dominant genre of theories in such literature is its foundation in the entrepreneurial organisations – a much narrower entity in comparison with Beck's unit of society. As a result, despite having provided a number of cues which go beyond its original source ultimately the source and the orientation it creates remain too strong. The problem also arises from the fact that both crisis and risk generically demand 'immediate' measures and accelerated actions, which go on to lend credibility to the toolkit approach.

The discussion here continues to emphasise the importance of the 'political' in more ways than one in the context of crisis communication and risk communication. Let me add that in a major way it also brings in the issue of surveillance. Though the next chapter will be solely devoted to this issue let me at this point refer to a scholar who has made a novel and pioneering effort in establishing a political link between risk with surveillance in these times. How the 'political' articulates itself in new modalities of intervention by integrating new mode of surveillance and new spaces of risk is analysed by Castel (1991:287–289) with lot of innovative clues. He refers to the rise of preventive policies in the contemporary times in which one does not start from a conflictual situation observable in experience, but does it by deducing it from a general definition of the dangers one wishes to prevent. He terms it as 'systematic predetection' and explains that in this form of surveillance the intended objective is that of anticipating and preventing the emergence of some undesirable event. But he adds an important dimension through the argument that this kind of surveillance dispenses with actual presence, contract and the reciprocal relationship of watcher and watched. This form, he notes, makes its presence 'in the flesh' or in short, on a certain form of individualisation. He also notes that it existed if only in the sublimated form of the observing gaze as a requisite of all the classic disciplinary, benevolent and therapeutic techniques, including Foucault's model of the panopticon. But a shift has taken place in the sense that thanks to the latest developments in technology surveillance can now be practised without any contact with, or even any immediate representation of, the subjects under scrutiny. Castel (p. 288) has this to offer in terms of greater clarity of the new mechanics at work:

> To intervene no longer means, or at least not to begin with, taking as one's target a given individual... What the new preventive policies primarily address is no longer individuals but factors, statistical correlations of heterogeneous elements. They deconstruct the concrete subject of intervention, and reconstruct a combination of factors liable to produce risk. Their primary aim is not to confront a concrete dangerous situation, but to anticipate all the possible forms of irruption of danger... To be suspected, it is no longer necessary to manifest symptoms of dangerousness or abnormality, it is enough to display whatever characteristics the specialists responsible for the definition of preventive policy have constituted as risk factors.

How crisis and risk are mutually implicated is a question that begs attention here. As we shall now see, the question is important in understanding their communicative dynamics. There are increasing efforts to explain the relationship and the frequency of such efforts is perhaps linked to the fact that both concepts are at centre stage of governing in disastrous times. Yet, describing the relationship in clear terms is not that easy. There is an interesting example of two scholars finding 'limitations' in their own description when faced with a crisis of bigger magnitude like health crisis. It leads them to look for clues in the peer descriptions of the relationship. Thus, for Sellnow and Seeger (2013:7–8) their own definition of crisis was that of a specific, unexpected, non-routine event or series of events creating high levels of uncertainty and a significant or perceived threat to high priority goals. This definition, they claim, captures the primary conditions of crisis and suggests that a crisis may be a contained, single event or it may be a series of interacting and cascading events. Their additional claim is that this definition also includes the idea that a crisis should be specific in its parameters. But having mentioned these points they are frank enough to admit that the larger issues like the ongoing healthcare crisis would not meet this definition. They sift through a number of perspectives on the issue but prefer to follow Heath's widely circulated 'straightforward' suggestion that a crisis is a risk manifested. Based on this perspective they point out that a risk occurs before a crisis and that crisis is the consequence of a risk continuing to develop without appropriate efforts to manage it. As they observe (p. 8), this notion of a risk 'incubating, developing unchecked, and perhaps interacting with other factors' is one of the most common views of a crisis "cause".' Risk communication, they further note, again relying on Heath, generally concerns 'risk estimates, whether they are appropriate, tolerable and risk consequences'. Another important point mentioned by them is that notwithstanding a general consensus about what constitutes a crisis there is almost always a debate about what, and who, caused a crisis. The problem assumes greater complications when communication is added to it. As they argue, it is because even if there may be a general consensus about communication ultimately being linked to the construction of meaning, sharing some interpretation or consensual understanding between senders/receivers, audiences, publics, stakeholders or communities, scholars widely differ on the locus of that meaning. With crisis and risk being so intimately connected in a complicated way it is not surprising that the locus issue also generates considerable debate concerning risk communication. The following set of questions raised by Chess et al. (quoted in Heath and Dan O'Hair, 2009:13) reveals why it is so:

> Is successful risk communication persuasion, transfer of information, public participation or empowerment of citizens to make decisions? Should it produce an informed citizenry, a compliant citizenry, an alert citizenry or an empowered citizenry? Should the goal be better decisions, fairer decisions, more consistent decisions, or, in the throes of environmental gridlock, any decisions at all? Or are there "different motivating forces" and therefore different risk communication goals, for every "group, person, agency administrator and middle manager"? These questions, in turn, have raised others about the ethics, and evaluation of risk communication.

The growing number of studies on crisis communication is apparently impressive, but one must take note of possible research gaps which lay themselves bare in grave situations caused by acute health crisis like the pandemic. Some scholars have been trying to warn the researchers about it for some time. Coombs (2009:115), for example, is one. He justifies the integral role of communication in crisis but argues that it is not a one-shot process as it concerns and adds value to the process of multiple negotiations of the pre-crisis, crisis response and post-crisis stages. He points out that at every stage communication is the lifeblood that fills the knowledge demands created by a crisis and allows people to make sense of it. In the process it also enables the collection, analysis and dissemination of crisis-related knowledge, thereby providing a foundation for decision-making. But the more important part of his observation concerns the mode of knowledge generation and its relatively peripheral attention in crisis communication research. He consults studies in crisis communication to identify and explain a lag in research focus that largely remains unaddressed in the otherwise proliferating literature – the intersection with knowledge. Coomb's view is that the limited research focuses on crisis communication has constrained what we could know about crisis communication, and that research that centres on crisis knowledge management is scant. He locates one reason for this neglect in the assumption that information is easy to collect, analyse, and disseminate, and this goes on despite the fact that the process is fraught with potential problems. This lag to a certain extent can be attributed to the techno-managerial orientation that continues to pervade health communication research in general. With some notable exceptions the toolkit approach avoids coming face-to-face with nagging uncertainties that pervade the complex terrain of epidemic/pandemic governance.

What goes on in the crisis communication research has a parallel in the risk communication research too. After reviewing literature on the H1N1 pandemic (2009–2011) and analysing the complexity and scale of current risk communication in the context of the governance of public health a group of researchers (Barrelet et al., 2013:119) identify three main research gaps. In each case they set a key question and provide the rationale:

i) How are risk perceptions dynamically influenced in an era of competing sources of information? Risk perceptions vary across time, social groups, cultures and countries. They are influenced by changing patterns of information gathering and dissemination (emergence of social media; competing sources of information; possible information overflow in some parts of the world). Trust building no doubt is a key aspect of risk perceptions. However, the critical variables that dynamically influence risk perceptions in a context of competing information sources have yet to be understood.
ii) How do competing narratives frame risk perceptions? Competing narratives (official statements and presentations, rumours, conspiracy theories, alternative worldviews and explanations, urban legends, hoaxes) about public health crises coexist in the public sphere to various degrees depending on the crisis. Their emergence patterns and relative impact on risk perceptions have yet to be understood.
iii) How do public health authorities manage to articulate risk communication theoretical principles and implementation, which carry scores of surprises?

They note that few studies report on how health authorities plan, develop and implement risk communication strategies. One cannot but agree with their contention that collection of such knowledge is important to foster learning through past experiences and organisational learning at all levels (international, national, local) and that it should include successes as well as past errors, misunderstandings, obstacles, shortcomings and public criticism related to risk communication.

The toolkit approach also remains completely oblivious to the cultural matrix of crisis communication and risk communication, and of health governance on a broader scale. As a result, it misses an important entry-point to garnering knowledge about crisis. In an innovative essay, making 'culture-centred interrogation' of health communication and outlining the potential scope of health communication scholarship, a study (Sastry and Dutta, 2017:10–14) draws attention among other things to the semiotic uncertainties of the infectious disease outbreaks. Citing the Ebola case it observes that significations around a disease – meanings, associations, risk, stigmas – are central in how the disease is understood, who is assigned responsibility (and blame), what resources are allocated and what solutions are considered. Consequently, it notes how the story of the crisis is told is of crucial importance to how the disease will progress and its human impact. Acknowledging the key role of communication but much like Coombs identifying the blind spot amidst the expanding literature, the study critically notes (p. 13), 'although the domain of meanings and social constructions of diseases is [sic] well within the provenance of communication scholarship, there is a curious lack of health communication theorizing on the socially constructed and ideological nature of categories like "outbreaks" or "emerging diseases" and the communicative premises of such articulations.'

When it comes to the chronicle of outbreak and its narrativisation Priscila Wald's book on *Contagious Cultures, Carriers, and the Outbreak Narrative* (2008) deserves some attention. She begins by referring to the WHO's global alert on the SARS outbreak in March, 2003, a crisis which has quite a few similarities with the COVID-19 outbreak. Each is a variety of the novel coronavirus, sharing Chinese provincial origin and having global spread. The two outbreaks also witnessed the similar response of epidemiologists exploring the possible sources of virus, media working 24×7 to inform public about the danger and medical researchers looking for the discovery of appropriate vaccine. Promising an 'evolving story of disease emergence' Wald finds (p. 2) in the successive accounts of 'emerging infections' a fascination not just with the novelty and danger of the microbes but also with the changing social formations of a shrinking world. She also confirms the presence of a dilemma during the pandemic times, which runs through this chapter in the form of a paradox, the simultaneity of the necessity and danger of human contact amidst 'profound sense of social interconnection' and 'communicability configuring community'. Describing contagion as 'more than an epidemiological fact', which rests much on social interactions and creation of social bonds Wald alludes to its basic instinct in terms of communicative dynamics when she observes that the circulation of microbes materialises 'the transmission of ideas'. She explicates (p. 3) the point this way:

> Outbreak narratives and *the* outbreak narrative have consequences. As they disseminate information, they affect survival rates and contagion routes. They promote or mitigate the stigmatizing of individuals, groups, populations, locales (regional and global), behaviours, and lifestyles and they change economies. They also influence how both scientists and the lay public understand the nature and consequences of infection, how they imagine the threat, and why they react so fearfully to some disease outbreaks and not others at least as dangerous and pressing. It is therefore important to understand the appeal and persistence of the outbreak narrative and to consider how it shapes accounts of disease emergence across genres and media globally.

Wald reconfirms her contention about the global impulse of outbreaks elsewhere (Wald's 'Foreword' in Nixon and Servitje, 2016:vii): Border-crossing microbes materialise the abstractions of contemporary geopolitics, manifesting the dangers and possibilities of the new connections, physical and metaphysical. As these microbes map the changing borders and relationships of a globalizing world, they are also vivid analogues for the mystical bonds of community. The scale of that community is variable: the outbreak narrative can mark the danger of strangers, hence reinforce the boundaries of the imagined community of the nation, for example or it can envision humanity united by their fragile humanity, their vulnerability, and, viscerally, by the contact illuminated by the circulating microbes, a mystically informed tactility.

Wald rightly finds in outbreak narratives the co-presence of the conventional and formulaic on the one hand, and its evolving nature on the other hand. One of her abiding concerns in the book is the (re)orientation of 'modernity' in outbreak times. Right from the beginning she intends to show how the depictions of impoverished spaces as 'primitive' temporalised the uneven development of global modernity and obscured the socioeconomic conditions of 'disease emergence'. On many occasions she also provides examples of how the rise of global paranoia and its politico-cultural dimensions threaten to disturb the multilevel interconnections of modernity. Consulting huge quantity of scientific, journalistic and mythic-fictional material of the twentieth and twenty-first centuries she contends that the outbreak narratives contain amplifications, dramatisations, myths and so forth on many fronts, including the ones generated by the mainstream media of various genres. At the end, she visualises in a tone of advocacy the possibility of revising the existing outbreak narrative to tell the story of disease emergence and human connection in the language of social justice rather than of susceptibility. Situating the outbreak narrative in the North–South continuum and 'human interconnections on a global scale' she has this suggestion to offer (p. 270):

> In place of the fearful scenario in which monstrous microbes from elsewhere threaten to turn "us" into "them" ("thirdworldification"), the revised story shows "thirdworldification" to be a product of uneven development and exploitation. Disease emergence, in this account, is an urgent problem in the North not only, or even primarily, because disease may spread from the South to the North, but because of the role of the North in perpetuating the conditions of thirdworldification worldwide. The inequities expressed by disease emergence make it imperative to address the conditions of poverty not chiefly because of the fear of contagion but because no human beings should have to live in the impoverished conditions that fuel the spread of disease. Communicable diseases are a part of life; they will continue to emerge and circulate, and people will suffer and die. Yet suffering and death should not be accepted as inevitable in one place and unthinkable in another.
>
> Amidst the uncertainties about the forecasted pandemic, there is no doubt that it, or any pandemic, will affect the world's populations inequitably. The emerging stories can exacerbate or begin to address the inequities.
>
> They can make a difference. It is not only possible but time to change the stories and the world they imagine.

Let me raise a basic question here: does community engagement or for that matter, crisis communication and risk communication matter much in governancing, especially when the neoliberal project has an uncompromising stand regarding the promotion of individualisation of responsibility? The question is not only related to the content of this chapter but with that of the whole volume. It is also inseparably linked with the recurring issue of having or not having to do with the 'political'. Considering the fundamental tenets of governance and its way of interpreting everything in terms of the profit-seeking market, access and quality of healthcare have been worst affected, with the state adopting 'austere' measures to rationalise the whole system in the name of efficiency and in the process lifting the 'safety net'. Neoliberalism, it is argued, has acquired epidemic proportions in the healthcare sector. Arguing why the contagion phenomenon should become a way to rethink the (western) liberal and neoliberal conceptualisations of autonomous, cordoned subjectivity Nixon and Servitje (2016:6) expose the guiding motive of healthcare reorganisation of the neoliberal project in a candid way:

> Today it is the lingering chronic illness, both figurative and metaphorical, that structures our cultural anxieties. The chronically ill citizen cannot contribute to a neoliberal society that prizes production, quotas, and stamina in the extreme social environment of the modern state that is increasingly devoid of social support for such "productivity". Making live and letting die become a question of calculating and calibrating endemicity and its effects. The victim of an *epidemic* disease, that is, at least functions in their death to relieve society of an unproductive member. The endemically ill linger and metaphorically contribute in the social imaginary to the troubling endemic conditions of "wasted energy" and "costs" which neoliberal actors seek to track, mitigate and eliminate both in and beyond traditional disciplinary structures of the school, the prison and the workplace.

If health, the foundation itself, is being reorganised in such terms 'community engagement' which is supposed to be formed and sustained with social capital (the 'inclination to do things for each other') as its motive force will be reset in ways that only resonate the political economic 'conditionalities' of governance. The neoliberal restructuring of the inequitable healthcare system is being analysed and critiqued in significant number of studies. Schrecker and Bramba (2015) associate the process with 'neoliberal epidemics'. They identify obesity, stress, austerity and inequality as four neoliberal epidemics and at the very outset unravel their political character by pointing out that that they are not only associated with but exacerbated by the rise of neoliberal politics. They are called epidemics because they make a quick transmission on an international scale across populations, and generate insecurity of all kinds by their very presence. Asserting (p. viii) that neoliberal politics has 'made us sick' they contemplate that had there been effective 'alternative' political and economic choices the dominance of neoliberal politics could have been prevented, or at least reduced, and we could have lived in a 'healthier' twenty-first century. The pessimistically coated account is balanced by their optimistically concluding note (p. 125) that neoliberal epidemics require a 'political cure' based on collectivism and solidarity. However, they stop there and do not stretch themselves to carve out a clear pathway to achieve such spirit. It may be due to the fact that the prevailing dominance of the neoliberal politics does not induce them enough to visualise it in a concrete form as yet.

Concluding remarks

The discussion above shows that health governance is a difficult terrain for negotiation and when linked to the pandemic it is becomes different ball game altogether for all. It is one thing to invoke 'community' and espouse the causes of 'engagement' theoretically and it is quite another to put such efforts in practice. The concept of community engagement in the health arena is not the same as it is in the case of say, forestry or academia/education (to refer to two major research themes of the community engagement literature) about which one can afford to go in a rather slow and steady manner. When a pandemic actually occurs all the hitherto neat step-by-step accounts of sensitising and mobilising communities are branded as 'utopian' and they tend to vanish almost instantly, firmly establishing reliance on the ready-reckoners. It also results in the concentration of power in the hands of the ruling forces. Such oligarchic concentration is initiated by governments adopting various strategies, sometimes crude, but in many cases subtle. The subtle strategies are invoked, as mentioned earlier, citing 'people's wellbeing'. But what is more important is that amidst an intense degree of collective anxiety, often bordering on the 'end of the world' panic, the monopolisation of power by few at the top may receive the approval of people. 'Democratic decision-making', quite a favourite expression of the theoretical proponents and practitioners of community engagement, loses its credence in grave crisis and the faith in the experts and specialists automatically goes up to an excessive degree. The avenues of participatory communication are closed down with top-down securitisation drives. As the COVID-19 outbreak has proved beyond doubt, leaving aside the authoritarian political systems which are based on a system of command and control, even in the widely recognised democratic polities health instantly becomes an issue about which people themselves begin to feel shy about speaking. The concentration of power thus is not only rationalised from above but also 'legitimated' at the bottom by those from whom the opportunities of articulation are taken away. In such cases communication acquires a linear flow, resurrecting its oldest but now discredited 'sender-message-channel-receiver' model. However, the greatest paradox of politics is that it does not let everything go one way in a totalistic manner. Linear communication may apparently seem to be effective for those who practise it, but it may lead to more complexities with some 'unintended consequences'. Hence, 'noise' in one form or the other is bound to remain and seek to subvert the dominant order of things even in pandemic times. The next and the last chapter will throw some light on it.

Notes

1 The notion of community has generated much literature over the centuries. Its extensive discussion is beyond the scope of this book. Accordingly, here after having introduced the notion in a general way, it is being mentioned in the specific context of community engagement, the main concern of the chapter.

2 Beck is well-known for making us aware of the twin phenomena of uncertainty and risk at the individual and community level, which he argues (Beck, 1992) are both an inevitable outcome and integral features of the modernity-led, technology-dependent society. For shifting uncertainty and risk from the margins of analysis to the centre stage he departed from the dominant path and theorised reflexive modernity (even using the term late modernity) to challenge the classical modernity's obsession with certainty and predictability. He has been called 'the prophet of uncertainty'. Beck has also been described (Tooz, 2020) as the 'pandemic intellectual' par excellence, with the comment that if he were alive he could have revealed startlingly new dimensions of the COVID-19 times marked by spiralling uncertainty and risk.

5

THE INFODEMIC SWITCH

Subversive communication

Introduction

It is only obvious that managing the COVID-19 pandemic is an exceptionally daunting task with multiple parameters, protocols, dimensions and phases. First and foremost, it involves managing people and reorienting existing material resources. Through numerous twists and turn it also involves at a later stage the tedious task of discovering or at least availing 'effective' vaccines. Even when that phase is over the next phase of building legitimacy and trust about the right kind of vaccines among diverse sections of people is equally tough. Together, the phases concern a complex combination of issues relating to science, technology, logistics and social psychological persuasion. In the absence of wider scientific literacy and robust health communication in most parts of the world, mis/disinformation tends to have free reign. As also mentioned a number of times in the preceding discussions, while there is a sustained effort in the pandemic times to enhance and concentrate power at the top of the governance hierarchy in different parts of the world its outcome is not totalistic; the reason being the non-linear nature of the multidimensional sources and channels of communication. The information flows have become so numerous that no force on earth, however powerful and ambitious, can have total control over them. It is noticeable that there has been a significant rise in infodemic (at times called 'disinfodemic' to put greater stress on negativity) with the escalation of the COVID-19 pandemic, when the virus and the virtual world come close and function in the mutual interest. At times it seems that the pace and reach of the infodemic surpasses those of the coronavirus, with lot of misleading consequences. The United Nations (United Nations Document, 2020) has also expressed grave concern about the intense growth of infodemic during the pandemic and the disregard for the international human rights standards and particularly the violation of the freedom of expression.

DOI: 10.4324/9781003247388-6

'Infodemic' mainly refers to the rapid spread of excessive quantity of misinformation and disinformation[1] of fake and false variety, though to a lesser degree it also involves accurate information. One major concern with infodemic is its tendency to make plausible and meaningful solutions to problems more and more elusive. This has obvious implications for governing in normal times and even more in non-normal times. Infodemic misleads the population, and as a kind of side effect it interferes with public's right to know and with the right of individuals to seek, receive and impart appropriate and credible information. Having particularly close relationship with health issues it received wide circulation since the severe acute respiratory syndrome (SARS) outbreak in 2003. In the COVID-19 context infodemic is explained in this chapter in a specific way, as a phenomenon marked by the coexistence and simultaneous operation of two contending processes of subversive communication:

i) Information creation, circulation and neutralisation by the tech giants having proprietorship of virtual platforms comprising social networking sites, social media[2] and search engines to exert control over the communication order.
ii) The seemingly countless users as sources utilising the power and reach of digital technology, which come in the way of unilateral dissemination of information from few sources.

It needs to be clarified at the outset that the overwhelming focus here on social media, the 'fifth estate' in the words of Mark Zuckerberg, the Facebook Chief Executive Officer, does not undermine the importance of the mainstream offline media. It is rather guided by the fact that in the contemporary times it is the social media which leads from the front and generates and controls for better or worse a surfeit of information. Social media has become a force to reckon with in the media ecosystem. Yet another point needs to be flagged here. Experience tells us that both governments and social media, two most powerful entities presently controlling our lives, lead as well as mislead. Accordingly, the discussion here will contain the argument that both the governments and the profit-seeking market forces make their own contributions to infodemic by indulging in disinformation, misinformation and inflated information. Infodemic goes on to serve commercial and political interests, often coalescing them in hitherto inconceivable ways vis-à-vis the state and non-state forces.

The pandemic meets mis/disinformation

With the coronavirus pandemic being what it is in terms of its spread and depth, it is only natural that the volume of information created and circulated by/with it would find no parallel. The two world wars had generated and circulated lot of information during their occurrence. With face-to-face communication, traditional media, snail mails, telephones and telegraphs as the mainstay of communication

– they also were marked by various instances of propaganda on either side, which inevitably involved mis/disinformation. But they were no match to the potpourri of of communication of the coronavirus infodemic and its two major propellers, media and new technology, in terms of structural inflation and cognitive penetration. Thanks to the astonishing progress of the cutting-edge information technology in particular the number of producers, disseminators and consumers of information in the contemporary times has assumed incredible proportions, far more than what could ever be imagined. Such development has been utilised to a bewildering extent by social media in particular. To refer to this large-scale transformation as a 'paradigm shift' is pertinent but perhaps not revealing enough unless and until one goes slightly deeper into the modus operandi of numerous actors and networks, and the angularities and nuances of the infodemic phenomenon. While I try do it in such extremely challenging circumstances the effort can at best be a modest one highlighting only certain key trends. No claim of having total knowledge of the backstage manoeuvring of the infodemic can be made. It is simply because the more one claims to have known more about it the more the terrain of the unknown expands. The paradox becomes graver with the 'uncomfortable' realisation that the burst of information does not necessarily lead to greater depth in meaning. On the contrary, it comes in the way of acquiring 'accurate and reliable' knowledge, obfuscating the transparency of communication of ideas, opinions and perspectives. The contemporary era is being widely described as the Information Age, the reason being that it facilitates the quantum of contact and engagement to an unprecedented extent. But the moot question is what kind of contact and engagement are being facilitated by it. The previous chapter revealed that collective/community engagement is a highly problematic affair, and that it is one thing to conceptualise it as an 'ideal' and another thing to realise it at the ground level. The same applies to communication, especially when it is sought to be interpreted in overwhelmingly 'social' (incorporating the 'political') terms over its technological and technocratic interpretations.

To refer back to the incidence of misinformation, the ongoing research on the theme has acquired increasing frequency in recent times, and more so with the coming of coronavirus. Based on a study of various 'claims' one study (Brennen et al., 2020:11) makes an inductive typology of the COVID-19-related misinformation and finds as many as nine points, which have relevance for the ensuing discussion in this chapter:

i) Public authority action/policy: such as, claims about state policy/action/communication, claims about the WHO guidelines and recommendations.
ii) Community spread: claims about the ways the virus is spreading internationally, in nations/states, or within communities. It also includes claims about people, groups or individuals involved/affected.
iii) General medical advice and virus characteristics: such as, health remedies, self-diagnostics, effects and signs of the disease.
iv) Prominent actors: claims about pharmacy companies or drug-makers, companies providing supplies to the healthcare sector, or other companies. Or,

claims about famous people, including those about which celebrities have been infected, about what politicians have said or done (but not if the misinformation is coming from politicians or other famous people).

v) Conspiracies: claims that the virus was created as a bioweapon, about who is supposedly behind the pandemic, and that the pandemic was predicted.
vi) Virus transmission: claims about how the virus is transmitted and how to stop the transmission, including cleaning, use of certain types of lights, appliances, protective gear and so forth.
vii) Explanation of virus origins: claims about where and how the virus originated (for example, in animals) and properties of the virus.
viii) Public preparedness: (normative) claims about hoarding, buying supplies, social distancing, (non)-adherence to measures and the likes.
ix) Vaccine development and availability: claims about vaccines, development and availability of a vaccine.

The researchers also categorise (p. 12) misinformation into the following: satire or parody; false connection (headlines, visuals or captions which do not support the content); misleading content (use of information to frame an issue or individual, when facts/information are misrepresented or skewed); false context (genuine content is shared with false contextual information, for example, real images which have been taken out of context); imposter content (genuine sources, for example, news outlets or government agencies, are impersonated); fabricated content (content is made up and cent percent false; designed to deceive and do harm); manipulated content (genuine information or imagery is manipulated to deceive, for example, deep fakes or other kinds of manipulation of audio and/or visuals).

A UNESCO-sponsored study (Posetti and Bontcheva, 2020:5) identifies four key disinfodemic formats:

i) Emotive narrative constructs and memes: false claims and textual narratives which often mix strong emotional language, lies and/or incomplete information, and personal opinions, along with elements of truth. These formats are particularly hard to uncover on closed messaging apps.
ii) Fabricated websites and authoritative identities: these include false sources, polluted datasets, and fake government or company websites, and websites publishing seemingly plausible information in the genre of news stories, for example, reporting bogus cases of COVID-19. The disinformation entailed can be shared by individuals, organised groups, some news media and official channels, wittingly or unwittingly. The disinfodemic often hides falsehoods among true information, and conceals itself in the clothes of familiar formats. It resorts to well-known methods, ranging from false or misleading memes and fake sources, to trapping people into clicking on links connected to criminal phishing expeditions. The result is that COVID-19 related disinformation affects contents across the board, including those about the origin, spread and incidence of the disease, symptoms and treatments and the responses from governments and other actors.

iii) Fraudulently altered, fabricated, or decontextualised images and videos: these are used to create confusion and generalised distrust and/or evoke strong emotions through viral memes or false stories.
iv) Disinformation infiltrators and orchestrated campaigns: aimed at sowing discord in online communities, advancing nationalism and geopolitical agendas, illicit collection of personal health data and phishing and monetary gain from spam and adverts for false cures.

These formats may also include artificial amplification and antagonism by bots and trolls as part of organised disinformation campaigns.

The above study also identifies (p. 6) nine prime themes of the disinfodemic:

i) Origins and spread of the coronavirus/COVID-19 disease: while scientists first identified cases of novel coronavirus (the virus that causes the disease) connected to an animal market in the Chinese city of Wuhan, there are many conspiracy theories pitting the blame on other actors and causes. The blame targets as different issues as the 5G network and chemical weapons manufacturers. It is added that using a label like 'Chinese virus' instead of neutral terminology inflates the location into an adjective, in an historical echo of early pandemics that gave a biased meaning to a noun.
ii) False and misleading statistics: often connected to the reported incidence of the disease and mortality rates.
iii) Economic impacts: the theme includes spreading false information about economic and health impacts of the pandemic, suggestions that social isolation is not economically justified, and even claims that COVID-19 is overall creating jobs.
iv) Discrediting journalists and credible news outlets: it is a theme often associated with political disinformation, with unsupported accusations that certain news outlets are themselves peddling in disinformation. This behaviour includes abuse levelled at journalists publicly but it is also used by less visible disinformation campaigns to undermine trust in verified news produced in the public interest. Attacks on journalists during the pandemic have been associated with crackdowns on critical coverage of political actors and states.
v) Medical science: symptoms, diagnosis and treatment: this theme includes dangerous disinformation about immunity, prevention, treatments and cures. For example, myriad 'sticky' memes claim that drinking or gargling cow urine, hot water or salt water could prevent the infection reaching lungs.
vi) Impacts on society and the environment: it ranges from panic buying triggers and false information about lockdowns to the supposed re-emergence of dolphins in Venetian canals.
vii) Politicisation: one-sided and positively-framed information is presented in an effort to negate the significance of facts that are inconvenient for certain actors in power. Other kinds of disinformation designed to mislead for gaining political advantage include: equating COVID-19 with flu; making baseless claims

about the likely length of the pandemic; and assertions about the (un)availability of medical testing and equipment.

viii) Content driven by fraudulent financial gain: it includes scams designed to steal people's private data.

ix) Celebrity-focused disinformation: this theme includes false stories about actors being diagnosed with COVID-19.

The Institute of Strategic Dialogue (ISD) in one of its briefing papers (ISD Policy Brief, 2020:1–14) has arrived at six key findings regarding the COVID-19 mis/disinformation campaign:

i) Both state-sponsored media and extremist movements are exploiting the situation to spread harmful and hateful messaging on social media.

ii) Anti-migrant and far-right networks are exploiting the situation to spread disinformation targeting migrants, refugees and other vulnerable populations online and offline as well as explicit threats of violence/harm to non-white populations from white supremacist groups online.

iii) Crisis points are playing into 'accelerationism' on the extreme right, which promotes the idea that democracy is a failure and that groups should accelerate its end through mobilising social conflict and violence.

iv) Misinformation about cures or treatments for coronavirus continue to circulate widely on Twitter and Facebook, often amplified by politicians and news media, and has contributed to fatal offline incidents.

v) Notwithstanding the technology platforms' efforts to address disinformation on COVID-19, platforms both large and small are hosting conspiracy theories. These theories may undermine efforts to deal with the crisis and its growth, including those disputing the reality of the virus and its impacts on health and life, which are particularly prevalent in closed groups and chat channels.

vi) There are some attempts to indulge in profiteering off the coronavirus pandemic through online platforms and advertising, despite platforms banning such practices.

Infodemic does not spare the WHO which claims to have taken the lead role in informing the world aware of the danger of the pandemic. In pandemic times it has been periodically issuing cautionary notes on the dangers of infodemic but it has itself come under extensive trolling and hate speech in the social media. It has been derisively described as the 'World Hoax Organisation', having been accused of generating misleading, conflicting and confusing messages on the crisis. However, its secretary general had mentioned, as early as in early 2020 before the coronavirus pandemic took place, the severity of the problem posed by the rising infodemic tide. In his speech in the Munich Security Conference (WHO Report III, 2020), held on 15 February, he had stressed the need to come together and face a 'common and dangerous enemy' with 'facts, not fear' and with 'rationality, not rumours'. The WHO's problem with the infodemic led him to be more forthright within months when he would assert (WHO Report IV, 2020) that that the situation warrants alongside the battle against the pandemic 'battling the trolls and conspiracy theorists that push misinformation and undermine the outbreak response'. Referring to the wide ranging misinformation and rumours involving food availability, remedial measures, immunisation and so forth he would also express concern that these are affecting even the best practices in the realm of public health. It is true that a major portion of the misinformation targets governments, public officials and international/transnational organisations, including the likes of the WHO. The policies and actions of such stakeholders must come under critical scrutiny during such public health emergency, but deliberate acts of misinformation have severely adverse impact on public perception. The 'Immunise the Public Against Misinformation' (WHO Report IV, 2020), a new UN alliance to fight the infodemic – comprising the WHO, UNESCO, International Telecommunication Union and UN Global Pulse – has received just over US $4.5 million from the COVID-19 Solidarity Response Fund to scale up its community amplifier work, social listening initiative, and other projects including the creation of a centralised fact-checking and misinformation centre to provide countries with appropriate tools to address the infodemic.

The WHO's initiatives to combat the infodemic includes the steps of developing global resources for fact-checking and misinformation management, infodemic measurement and analysis, evidence synthesis, knowledge translation, risk communication, community engagement and fabrication of messages. It is noteworthy, especially in the context of the previous chapter, that both risk communication and community engagement are part of the strategisation of 'sharing information responsibly'. Incidentally, in partnership and alliance build-up the WHO has accorded much importance to monitoring and collaborating with social media and social networking platforms such as Facebook, Google, Tencent, Baidu, Twitter, TikTok, Weibo, Pinterest, which are the key players in both facilitating and (supposedly) countering the infodemic. Reflecting on the dysfunctional impact of the relationship between the prevailing infodemic and misinformation a document (PAHO-WHO Factsheet, 2020:1) notes the following:

> Misinformation is false or inaccurate information deliberately intended to deceive. In the context of the current pandemic, it can greatly affect all aspects of life, especifically [sic] people's mental health, since searching for COVID-19 updates on the Internet has jumped 50%–70% across all generations. Misinformation in a pandemic can negatively affect human health. Many false or misleading stories are fabricated and shared without any background or quality checking. Much of this misinformation is based on conspiracy theories, some introducing elements of these into seemingly mainstream discourse. Inaccurate and false information has been circulating about all aspects of the disease: how the virus originated, its cause, its treatment and its mechanism of spread. Misinformation can circulate and be absorbed very quickly, changing people's behavior, and potentially leading them to take greater risks. All this

> makes the pandemic much more severe, harming more people and jeopardizing the reach and sustainability of the global health system.

Also noting (p. 2) that misinformation expands at the same pace as content production and distribution paths grow and this in turn contributes simultaneously to the acceleration of infodemic it mentions five ways in which the process takes effect:

i) Making it hard for people, decision makers and health workers to find trustworthy sources and reliable guidance when they need it. Sources may be apps, scientific organisations, websites, blogs, 'influencers', and more.
ii) People may be feeling anxiety, depression, overwhelmed, emotionally drained and unable to meet important demands.
iii) Possibility of affecting decision-making processes when immediate answers are expected, and not enough time is allotted to deeply analyse the evidence.
iv) Having no quality control on what is published, and sometimes, on what is used to take action and make decisions.
v) Possibility of anyone writing or publishing anything on the web (podcasts, articles, etc.), in particular on social media channels (individual and institutional accounts).

It needs to be clarified that several organisations like the WHO and PAHO are periodically coming out with communication planning and guidelines on epidemics, especially since the beginning of this century. The literature was germinating slowly but it began to gather momentum and consolidate since 2005, in the aftermath of the SARS pandemic. The pre-COVID-19 literature is important because it had set the ball rolling in making the world aware that not just the infodemic but also its operation in the particular context of health emergencies has the potential not only to cause panic, paranoia, social disorder and chaos, but also to endanger the lives of many.

But nothing seemed to have matched the frequency and quantity of literature on the coronavirus infodemic. It has many strands but one major strand, as already noted, constitutes the conspiracy theories, which are constructed and disseminated with alarming speed and intended to intensify negativity among people. It is no wonder that such theories have attracted the attention of researchers. Thus, describing coronavirus as the 'king of disinformation' a study (Krekó and Szicherle, 2020) lists four groups of such theories prevalent in the fake news framework: the first group consists of 'genocide theories' suggesting that someone is deliberately spreading the virus intentionally to achieve a certain goal. It notes that the 'most typical narrative' in this group claims that the 'global elite' – including Bill Gates – is seeking to decimate the population of the earth. The second group includes the 'biological weapon theories'. Typical theories in this group claim that a biological weapon is being used against China in a 'Third World War'. One specific narrative of this category claims, for instance, that the US is behind the outbreak to 'bring the Chinese economy to its knees'. This narrative, it is observed, fits perfectly into the well-known geopolitical narrative often disseminated by Russia and China that suggests the US acts in a hostile manner against all of its perceived rivals, even if it means breaking international conventions. The study also observes another 'suggestion' in this category, which is by far one of the most familiar ones – that the virus was spread by China, and it was created as a biological weapon in a military lab in Wuhan. The claim is that the coronavirus is not something that occurred naturally, but is a result of a specific plan aiming to annihilate a group of people. The third group of disinformation consists of the apocalyptic 'end of the world' narratives. In this case the narratives 'seek sensation with claims that can sow panic.' There were claims about a civil war in Wuhan, supposing that hundreds of infected people 'besieged' checkpoints leading out of the area, and even that almost 5 million people had left Wuhan, thereby fanning the assumption that the virus has already spread throughout the world. The fourth group consists of articles about 'cures', based on the wishful pieces stating that an antidote to the virus has been found in the form of a processed version of traditional Chinese medicine and also in the form of a miracle 'cure' in Vitamin C. More instances of mis/disinformation will be cited as the discussion proceeds.

The above study also expresses some concern about clickbait publications and their role in spreading disinformation. The introductory part of this chapter mentions the role of the profit-seeking market forces vis-à-vis the rise of the infodemic. There will be more discussion on it subsequently in the specific context of social media, but clickbait publications may be referred here. Not easy to notice, a development in the pandemic times is the steady growth of clickbait pages and write-ups thematically dealing with the virus and its possible effects. The rise of such publications has long-term implications. This aspect, not much in the limelight mainly due to its 'hidden' modus operandi, merits some mention, howsoever brief. Clickbait is basically an emerging digital marketing technique of increasing importance, primarily used to drive page views on websites. The motive is to attract viewership for some intrinsic purposes, particularly to push an opinion or a view and blend it with procuring online advertising revenue. It is argued (Issak and Hanna, 2020:58) that with real-time monitoring of advertising responses on targeted individuals, including real-time substitution to find 'click bait' that worked, the advertising campaign is able to both maximise its impact and detect trends not visible at the macro scale. On occasions there may also be the motive of making phishing attacks to spread malicious files or steal user information. The COVID-19 pandemic being a great source of information manipulation for commercial and political profit-seeking clickbait pages and write-ups scale up their presence and importance in the infodemic scene.

It is only natural that there will be intense deliberations and debates on the downsides of infodemic and the fate of mis/disinformation, and they would continue for a long time. Nor is it surprising that the experts taking part in such debates would be a divided lot, with one side forecasting a decline in mis/disinformation and the other side arguing that it will intensify in the coming decade. After studying such debates, centring around a survey of technologists, scholars, practitioners, strategic thinkers and others, two analysts (Anderson and Rainie, 2017) find the respondents 'evenly split' on the following query: in the next ten years, will trusted methods emerge to block false narratives and allow the most accurate information to prevail in the overall information ecosystem? Or will the quality and veracity of information online deteriorate due to the spread of unreliable, sometimes even dangerous, socially destabilising ideas? They point out (pp. 3–5) that broadly those forecasting improvement place their hopes in technological fixes and in societal solutions while the other side assert that the dark side of human nature, especially of 'bad actors with bad motives', is aided and not stifled by technology. Interestingly, the study refers to an online canvassing survey of 2017, which reveals almost a 'tie' with 49% respondents being optimistic about a better information environment and 51% being pessimistic and forecasting a further decline in it. The latter study explains that those experts who are hopeful tend to believe that 'technology can help fix these problems', the argument being that the rising speed, reach and efficiencies of the Internet, apps and platforms can be harnessed to rein in fake news and misinformation campaigns. Some would predict that better methods will in course of time arise to create and promote trusted, fact-based news sources. There is another strand in such optimism. It is also stressed that it lies in human nature to come together and fix problems, that people have always adapted to change and that this current wave of challenges will also be overcome. The related point is that misinformation and bad actors have always existed but they have eventually been marginalised by well-meaning and smart people and processes. The optimists expect that well-meaning actors will work together to find ways to enhance the information environment for betterment and that better information literacy among citizens will enable people to judge the veracity of material content and eventually raise the tone of discourse. The pessimists base their contention on two cardinal points. First, the fake news ecosystem preys on some of our deepest human instincts. It means that the primal quest of human beings is for success and power and that their 'survival' instinct will continue to degrade the online information environment in the next decade. They predicted that manipulative actors would use new digital tools to take advantage of inbred preference of human beings for comfort and convenience and their craving for the answers they find in reinforcing echo chambers. Second, the brains of human beings are not wired to contend with the pace of technological change. The argument here is that the rising speed, reach and efficiencies of the Internet and the emerging online applications will magnify these human tendencies and that technology-based solutions will not be able to overcome them. In this case the visualisation is that of a future information landscape in which fake information crowds out reliable information. Some pessimists even foresaw a world in which widespread information scams and mass manipulation cause broad swathes of public to simply give up on being informed participants in civic life.

My own stance on this issue is that given the overall global political scenario as scripted by the state-market (corporate) collaboration the infodemic and the 'disinformation society' are issues which involve but go beyond the question of mis/utilisation of information technology. It is more a question of the concerned actors who pull the strings from behind to run the show in which the cutting-edge technology is only a serving tool. This stance makes it unavoidable that the virtual platform, with special reference to social media, is to be brought under the purview of the discussion.

Platform politics and social media

In recent times academic writings on the growing importance and networking of platform society, platform economy and platform governance are becoming more and more evident. Even if it is not always articulated directly the implicit mechanism that is at work in such conceptual developments is the platformisation of information. There are studies (such as Dijck et al., 2018) which specifically identify datafication and commodification as the two foundation pillars of the platformisation of news, along with quantified audience and curated content as key features of the platform ecosystem in the connective world. 'Health' is detected as one of the main issues for manoeuvring the coming of the platform ecosystem. It hardly needs to be pointed out that health crisis provides greater scope for more extensive and intensive manoeuvring. The astonishing development of new technology enhanced the scope further. During the pandemic times quarantine and social distancing have resulted in an exponential rise in digital proximity. It has created a 'digitise or die' dictum in a subtle but radical form. The pandemic provided the big tech corporations a huge boost as part of a tectonic shift towards a 'no-touch' future (Klein, 2020). This has led to the rise of the platform politics in which virtual platforms, social networking sites, social media and search engines play an aggressive role in repackaging information and knowledge in their own terms. The traditional media would lag behind in the race in terms of both access and usage, and the win–win situation is exclusively reserved for social media. Social media is composed of interactive forms of electronic communication through which users create online communities to share information, ideas, personal messages, and other content and through which they can share, co-create, discuss, participate and modify user-generated content or self-curated content posted online. Social media, having a steady growth since 2004–2006, witnessed a dramatic expansion in usage during the pandemic. According to one account (Data Sheet I, 2020), as of July, 2020, more than 3.96 billion people use social media, which equals nearly 51% of the global population. The annual growth in the total number of social media users is 10.5%, which in terms of number is more than 376 million. Before the focus is shifted towards a qualitative assessment of its functions and role it may be appropriate to mention some data (Data Sheet II, 2020) about the phenomenal rise of the latest but arguably the most potent variety of media. Facebook, launched in 2004, has daily active users to the tune of 1.6 billion and 2.4 billion monthly active users. It is the largest social network in the world. Facebook video has approximately 8 billion video views per day. YouTube, established in 2005, has daily active users to the tune of 149 million and 1.9 billion monthly active users. YouTube has 5 billion views per day. On average 300 hours of video are uploaded every minute on YouTube. WhatsApp, formed in 2009, has 1 billion daily active users, 1.5 billion monthly active users and 60 billion messages sent every day. Established in 2010, Instagram has 600 million daily active users and 1 billion monthly active users. There are now 500 million daily stories users. Since its creation, more than 40 billion photos have been shared. On average 95 million photos are uploaded daily on Instagram. There are approximately 4.2 billion likes per day. Twitter, founded in 2006, has more than 330 million monthly active users and 134 million daily active users. The daily new accounts opened reach 460,000 and daily new tweets are close to140 million. Each twitter user has on an average 208 followers. 550 million accounts are reported to have at least sent a tweet. Reddit, founded in 2005, has approximately 330 million monthly active users. It is estimated that it gets over 14 billion views per month. There have been more than 853,000 subreddits. It has more than 138,000 active communities. On average there are 25 million votes on Reddit daily. LinkedIn, founded in 2002 and launched in 2003, has over 560 million registered users. It is estimated that it has approximately 303 million monthly active users. 5.3 million new accounts per month are created on it. There are over 30 million company pages. Snapchat, established in 2011, has approximately 301 million monthly active users. It also reports 109 million daily active users. It is competing closely with its rival, Facebook, by reporting more than 10 billion video views daily. Approximately 3 billion snaps are created every day. It is estimated that it would take one person more than 950 years to watch all snaps made in a day. Pinterest, founded in 2010, has 291 million monthly active users. The total number of Pinterest pins is more than 175 billion. The total number of Pinterest boards is approximately 1 billion. In a day, Pinterest is visited by 2 million users, who save shopping pins on their boards.

Social media is not going away, and it is to contribute to the information ecosystem more than ever before. Having brought an unprecedented opportunity to let common people exchange information and communicate among themselves and by facilitating groupthink it could not but be so. Its origin is much different from that of the conventional mainstream media, and as the following comment Chambers, 2020:5) shows, its importance as the source and circulation of'important facts' was more of an 'unintended consequence':

> Social media came into the world not as an organ of the free press, not as news and information services, not as the mediator between citizen and state, and not even as a mediator between citizens and citizen, but as a fun way for people to socialize (and, it turns out, a good way to make money). Their epistemic role and function as transmitters of important facts about what is going on the world, including the world of politics, was an unintended development. Perhaps this role could have been predicted, but it is not what they were designed, or apparently prepared, for.

The comment is valid if one considers the history of origin of social media. However, the fact is that generating an innovative and spectacular dynamics it has been able to transform the 'unintended consequence' into an inevitable process. Things have come to such a pass that not just in normal times but also in times of emergencies its 'vital' role is being acknowledged. Theorists of crisis communication have recognised the role of social media in clear terms and the following excerpt (Sellnow and Seeger, 2013:131) is an instance:

> The application of new social media or Web 2.0 technologies…increases the speed and richness of information shared across and within the groups. Of special interest is the information generated by the public and shared with others in the public space. (T)he public is already using social media to share and modify information. The increasing use of social media by the public during crises and disasters puts the public now at the center of a crisis and disaster, conveying important information and response needs.

There is, however, more to the twin processes of 'sharing and modifying' than meets the eye. As a prelude to a more elaborate discussion it may be observed that social media in general and more so in times of crisis plays a dual role laced with highly contradictory impulses. Borrowing from Robert Louis Stevenson's classic piece it can be explained as the Dr Jekyll and Mr Hyde syndrome. On the one hand, infodemic has a positive role in democratising both access and use of information by involving numerous people in the communication loop. On the other hand, in a negative stroke such wider participation of creators-disseminators-users vis-à-vis informational flow results in the circulation of an unimaginable and uncountable quantity and wide variety of rumours, fake news, false data and so forth. The barrage of mis/disinformation in the communication ecosystem is both top-down and bottom up, the first category relates to the flow from the traditional influencers like politicians, officials, experts, advisers, celebrities and prominent public figures to the people, and the second concerns the flow from the people 'down below'. An ample scope of retaining anonymity and false identity has enhanced the subversive potential of social media to an enormous degree. There is no doubt that with the coming of social media the common people for the very first time have a technological tool at their disposal, which puts them in three simultaneous roles of producers, disseminators and consumers in the communication loop. The twin processes of 'popularisation' and 'democratisation' of mediation have shaken the traditional grammar of the communication ecosystem in a manner which seems near-irreversible, at least at this moment.

The most challenging impact of the development has been on the status of 'factual' information. There are facts existing all around us but the ways mis/disinformation has repackaged them with bias and falsehood make it extremely difficult to confidently distinguish fact from fiction. The frequency and pace with which such packaging is done far exceed that of fact-checking by few dedicated media watch organisations. The COVID-19 pandemic has resulted in the free play of mis/disinformation because much about the virus being unknown and unpredictable there is a race for making everything known and predictable in any which way one can. Yet, when facts themselves are being targeted for profit-seeking fact-checking cannot be an easy exercise by any means. It not only involves the tedious task of identifying mis/disinformation but also coming in the way of extremely powerful corporations and governments which manipulate data and information to serve their interests. It does result in repressive measures by governments and by these corporate forces. Then there is also the sensitive question of the credibility of the watchdog organisations themselves. At a more abstract level, while the fact-checkers are supposed to make their regulatory contribution to 'accurate' and 'reliable' knowledge what is 'fact' is itself a very dicey issue in the world. It is so not the least because of the confusing yet increasing scepticism about the definition and legitimacy of 'fact' itself but also because of the consequent argument in favour of the 'relativity' of facts. The root of the problem and complexity with the indeterminacy of 'fact' lie with the challenging position faced by 'truth'. Itself. As Bernard Williams explains (2002:1), together with the demand for truthfulness there is the 'equally pervasive suspicion about the truth itself, involving whether there is any such thing or whether it can be relative or subjective or something of that kind.' A study (Seaton et al., 2020) explores the root of the problem in the fact-checkers themselves, notwithstanding their commitment to protect democratic systems from the avalanche of false information, inflamed feelings and widely-believed conspiracies. They are stated to have found themselves 'willy-nilly in the middle of a bewildering new information revolution' characterised by the global problem of 'bad information'. The study concentrates on the COVID-19 pandemic and asserts that it has made fact-checking much harder. It explains (p. 2) how the information game is made more complicated by the virus:

> What we discover about COVID-19, how it spreads, to whom and why, and how best to mitigate it – all depend on information. Yet, the virus has exploited fissures in societies and raced through vulnerabilities left by pre-existing inequality. It has exposed what we knew but had chosen to ignore. How we individually, collectively, socially, politically, and internationally cope with it depends on what we know and how we understand it. Previous pandemics were often managed by great infrastructural developments: sewers and clean water for cholera; draining marshes and living in cities for malaria; and this one will require a new infrastructure settlement, but this time it will be of information, not materials.

The most decisive effect of the development depicted here has been the realisation that it is not that easy to drive out 'stupid', 'wrong' and 'bad' information by good information.

The tsunami of mis/disinformation in the pandemic times took off quite early, as early as in March, 2020. It started covering wide ranging issues, including the virus' place of origin and source, its nature, diagnosis procedures, cures or preventative measures or treatments, emergency responses, funny or feel-good stories, social misbehaviour, number of deaths, politicians' responses, the first reported cases and various other activities. Let me present some samples presented by the Centre for Informed Democracy and Social Cyber Security (IDeaS, 2020). The samples are not exhaustive but they are substantially indicative of the range of mis/disinformation pervading the social media: there is no coronavirus, the virus is a normal flu and is not much dangerous, the virus was leaked from the Wuhan Institute of Virology in China, gargling with bleach will be the prevention/cure, spraying chlorine on body prevents the virus, drinking cow urine and applying cow dung on the body can lead to cure, Asians are more likely to get the virus, Africans are immune, everyone with COVID-19 dies, washing hands is a marketing propaganda by soap companies, all human interactions need to be stopped to prevent the spread of the virus, if one can hold one's breath for ten seconds one does not have the virus, one month of social distancing stops the epidemic permanently, constant sex kills the virus, the pandemic and the lockdown caused cleansing of Venice's waterways to enable swans and dolphins to return and take over, Saddam Hussein in the 1990s had informed his cabinet of the US threat to spread coronavirus if its command was not followed, Russia unleashed over 500 lions to compel people stay indoors amidst the outbreak, the Chinese coronavirus patients are being cremated alive, riots taking place in London due to unavailability of food during the lockdown and martial law being imposed there, the municipality in Bengaluru in India spraying medicine in the air to kill the virus, Kenya hiring the Maasai tribesmen to enforce lockdown, the Indian police beating up street children defying lockdown, people in India beating up the police for enforcing lockdown, restaurants owned by Muslims in Bengaluru spreading the virus by spitting in food, the Hindus dropping religious statues in sea because they are found to be useless in COVID-19 crisis and so forth. Some of the items here are satirical, some funny and hilarious, some clearly absurd, some atrocious and scandalous, some racist, some downright contradictory, some complementary to each other, but many of them are highly dangerous if taken seriously, and many surely have the potential to aggravate the crisis and disrupt the order needed to tackle it. A study by Li et al. (2020), exploring the dissemination of misinformation through YouTube, finds that over one-quarter (27.5%) of the most viewed YouTube videos on COVID-19 contained misleading information, reaching millions of viewers worldwide. The study recommends that as the pandemic worsens public health agencies must better use YouTube to deliver timely and accurate information and to minimise the spread of misinformation and play a significant role in successfully managing the pandemic. It also notes that YouTube has been a significant source of misleading information during the earlier public health crises, including the H1N1, Ebola and Zika outbreaks. In those cases it was found that approximately 23% to 26% of YouTube videos were misleading, while videos from reputable sources were vastly under-represented. Apart from the usual fare of racist, discriminatory remarks the study also refers (p. 5) to an interesting piece of conspiracy theory, which is as follows: The world is controlled by a cult. This cult wants to control everyone. These people are the 1% and use an underground force to control people. This cult uses the mainstream media to tell premade versions of a story in order to incite fear and control in the public. Coronavirus is an example of one of these control tactics. This is done to control the economy to destroy small business.

Elusive control

The struggle to minimise the impact of the infodemic goes on. A document (UNESCO Issue Brief I, 2020:4) mentions various strategies through which social media, social networking sites and search engine companies seek to address the infodemic:

i) Content moderation: removing, down ranking or labelling COVID-19 disinformation. This is increasingly done through automated systems powered by Artificial Intelligence (AI). However, it also entails some problems. Thus, sometimes legitimate expression may be caught in the Net, and wrongly identified and taken down.
ii) Soliciting donations to fact-checkers and journalists so that the experts can carry on the task of countering mis/disinformation with adequate funding.
iii) Directing the users towards official health information sources created by partnering with national and international public health organisations (including WHO) and through information centres formally in charge of official information. Steps are being taken to optimise such information at the top of news feeds or in search results.
iv) Advertising policies: a number of companies have banned advertisements that include COVID-19 disinformation but it is still inadequate as there are people online able to peddle falsehoods for profit.

Incidentally, the document has an interesting depiction (p. 12) of mis/disinformation and of the protecting role of free press as a countering entity: 'Information is the air you breathe, lies are like the virus, and a free press is the mask.'

At a later stage infodemic has targeted vaccines too. The Royal Society (2020:1–35) in a collaborative paper with the British Academy (p. 6) has expressed apprehension about vaccine deployment facing 'information mixed with fear and rumour with the rise of misinformation that fills knowledge voids under conditions of uncertainty.' It results in the decline in the three essential elements of 'vaccine confidence' – importance, safety and effectiveness. A research report (Rory et al., 2020:1–96) of the English, Spanish and Francophone social media reflects a strong concern about the complexity of the vaccine information ecosystem in which a 'cacophony of voices and narratives', reinforced by unreliable information and misinformation, coalesce to create an 'environment of extreme uncertainty'. The report identifies the interplay of political and economic motives of actors and institutions involved in vaccine development and the safety, efficacy and necessity concerns around vaccines. It finds many instances of online vaccine conversations and narratives exacerbating mistrust in the intentions of institutions and key figures surrounding vaccines. There is also reference to the growing number of 'data deficits', implying high demand for information about a topic combined with low supply of credible information, being exploited by 'bad actors' to complicate efforts of invention of vaccines. The concern leads to the observation (p. 6) that we have reached a 'pivotal and hypersensitive crossroads where increasing rates of vaccine skepticism may not only jeopardize the effectiveness of a potential COVID-19 vaccine, but that of vaccines more broadly, and even levels of trust in institutions connected to science and medicine.' to a certain extent, the observation has come true by the end of 2020, when one finds news (The Economist, 2020) of the activities of anti-vaxxers and arguments favouring rejection of the invented COVID vaccines, which emerged in European countries like France, Italy, Poland and Hungary. In some cases even the political leaders are intensifying the vaccine scepticism. An apparently comic but potentially dangerous portent (The Indian Express, 2020) in making a serious issue too light came from the Brazilian President, Jair Bolsonaro, who cautioned the citizens that his government will not be responsible if the Pfizer/BioNTech vaccine turns people into 'crocodiles' or make women bearded as a side effect. (Incidentally, his wife defied him and got herself vaccinated.) One interesting recommendation in the research report (p. 75) is to stop relying on fact-checking efforts and platforms' content moderation policies to address data deficits. The logic of such unconventional path is that actions like fact-checking and content moderation are reactive, insufficient and potentially counterproductive. It is further explained that greater levels of content moderation could fuel anti-vaccination narratives that claim that platforms are attempting a cover-up, and it could also encourage key vaccine communities to migrate to alternative platforms that are harder to monitor and research. Thus, preference is expressed for proactive messaging that is both compelling and tailored to different audiences.

None would doubt that such proposals and measures are needed to stem the free play of the infodemic. If the efficacy of the vaccines is to be doubted it must be done scientifically and not on the basis of mis/disinformation. There can be more such proposals and measures to counter mis/disinformation not only in the pandemic times but even in 'normal' times, considering the dubious role of the infodemic. However, a fundamental problem with such efforts to counter the flip side of the infodemic is that they have a tough task in confronting the reality in which both the governments and the corporate forces take advantage of the situation and cooperate with each other, often taking advantage of the power of social media. Hence, one would find instances of both the governments and the major stakeholders of social media issuing ethical messages favouring 'accurate', 'reliable' and even (the practically impossible) 'neutral' presentation of information, along with the so-called community guidelines – all laced with the appeal and/or self-declaration of 'strict adherence' to the same. But it does not need much effort to find out that there are times when the preachers themselves violate their own terms and become the perpetrators. The increasing collaboration between the state/government and the corporate forces, in which the mainstream media in general and the social media in particular are the beneficiaries, ensures that such violations of rules go unnoticed by the respective parties, or that indifference is shown even when they are brought to their notice, except only on occasions when the respective interests of government and the corporate forces directly collide with such violations.

Considering its reach and power as one of the most potent forces shaping the mediated reality, let me refer to the community guidelines issued by the Instagram (Instagram Community Guidelines, 2020), now under the ownership of the most powerful of them all, Facebook. The guidelines begin with the assurance that in the times of 'unprecedented public health emergency' Instagram wants to ensure that an updated version serves to protect people from the harmful content and 'new types' of abuse related to COVID-19. It is asserted that Facebook is working hard to remove content that has the potential to contribute to real-world harm, including through our policies prohibiting coordination of harm, sale of medical masks and related goods, hate speech, bullying and harassment and misinformation that contribute to the risk of imminent violence or physical harm.

There is also a promise that the organisation would continue to look at the content on the platform, assess speech trends, and engage with experts and will provide additional policy guidance when deemed appropriate. The short-term guidelines are to post only one's own photos and videos, consistence obedience to the law, and not to indulge in spamming or posting nudity. The long-term category concerns the claim that being a reflection of diverse community of cultures, ages and beliefs Instagram makes efforts to create a safe and open environment for everyone, but with provisions for deleted content, disabled accounts or other restrictions. It is also claimed that Facebook, in some cases, allows content for public awareness which would otherwise go against its community guidelines. It supposedly does so if the concerned material is found newsworthy and in public interest, but there is the assurance that it would be done only after weighing the public interest value against the risk of harm, and keeping in mind the international human rights standards.

The more concrete stipulations, bordering on a plan of action, include the following:

i) Share only photos and videos that one has taken or has the right to share. Posting of authentic content, and not the one's copied or collected from the Internet.
ii) Posting photos and videos that are appropriate for a diverse audience. Nudity in photos of paintings and sculptures are permitted but no other forms of portrayal of nudity are allowed. In this regard special attention is claimed to be provided to the portrayal of women and children.
iii) Fostering meaningful and genuine interactions. It involves discouraging the following items: artificially collecting likes, followers or shares, posting repetitive comments or content, or repeatedly contacting people for commercial purposes without consent from the concerned sources; monetary transactions in exchange for likes, followers, comments or other engagement; content that engages in, promotes, encourages, facilitates or admits to the offering, solicitation or trade of fake and misleading user reviews or ratings; inaccurate information; impersonation of accounts.
iv) Follow the law. It is asserted that Instagram is not a place to support or praise terrorism, organized crime, or hate groups.
v) Respecting other members of the Instagram community. Fostering a positive, diverse community and removing content that contains credible threats or hate speech, content that targets private individuals to degrade or shame them, personal information meant to blackmail or harass someone, and repeated unwanted messages. Stronger conversation is allowed around people who are

featured in the news or have a large public audience due to their profession or chosen activities but there is resistance to encouraging violence or attacking anyone on the basis of race, ethnicity, national origin, sex, gender, gender identity, sexual orientation, religious affiliation, disabilities or diseases. However, there is a qualifier: when hate speech is being shared to challenge it or to raise awareness, it may be allowed, if there is clear expression of the intent. Serious threats of harm to public and personal safety are not allowed. This includes specific threats of physical harm as well as threats of theft, vandalism and other financial harm. It is added that there is a careful review of the reports of threats and many points are considered in determining whether a threat is credible.

vi) Maintaining the supportive environment by not glorifying self-injury. Among other things like eating disorders there is also a specific mention of the removal of content identifying victims or survivors of self-injury if the content targets them for attack or humour.

vii) Being thoughtful when posting newsworthy events. It involves the possibility of removing videos of intense and graphic violence to ensure appropriate platform for everyone. It is also clarified that if such contents are shared to condemn, raise awareness or educate one has to provide photo caption with a warning about graphic violence. However, sharing graphic images for sadistic pleasure or to glorify violence is ruled out.

In mid-April, 2020, Facebook stated its intention to let the users know if they have spread 'bad information'. It was to let them know if they liked, reacted to or commented on posts with harmful misinformation about coronavirus, which were removed. Moreover, the process included directing the users engaged with those posts to avail information on virus myths debunked by the WHO. Facebook also banned bogus advertisements promising coronavirus treatments or cures as 'no such thing exists'. It claims that its algorithms are being altered, and through an information page efforts are being made to put before users the facts about the virus from global health organisations and from the health departments at state and local levels. Tinkering with algorithms is not necessarily a viable solution though and the reasons will be explained below.

There is no doubt that mis/disinformation has a much faster speed and much like the virus itself it has an astonishing capacity of mutation, which seem to have made the preventative measures, even the most updated ones, less than adequate. There are models which show that fake news moves six times faster than true news. The 'winning side' is aided by the 'massification' of information technology around the world. The infodemic factor during the pandemic has also brought to the fore another issue which has already been there but in a less visible way: that the steeper control of new technology and media with increasing number of regulations will hamper the growth and sustenance of the communication ecosystem and facilitate the oligarchical rule of the statist and the market forces, and lack of effective control mechanism will tilt the infodemic even more towards mis/disinformation. The basic problem is that no one has a definite clue about the optimum point, if it at all exists.

This is perhaps disconcerting but not surprising if one remembers that the line between freedom and control has been perennially blurry. One can even go further to note that the demarcation is even more indistinct when it concerns the freedom of expression. The extreme point of tension between freedom of expression and control is reached in situations of emergencies, including health emergencies. The UNESCO description, mentioned above, of the free press as the 'mask' in the sense of being a secure and protective gear, sounds quite impressive and desirable but in a world dominated by the mainstream corporate media conglomerates it remains, barring some exceptional instances of critical articulations here and there, a utopia constrained by a dystopia in the form of infodemic. Freedom of expression is only achievable when it is socialised at the base to assume an organic form. Social media being a game changer in the global context could have theoretically facilitated such process but witnessing its modus operandi one realises that mere romanticisation of its 'social' character in the sense of it becoming a tool of articulation of common people may as well result in the struggle for free and fair access to media going many steps backwards. Then again, all this brings us to the highly complicated, sensitive and tenuous relations between the mediated reality and critical discourse of democracy, which demands a more extensive analysis than what can be offered here. It may sound a bit dramatic but there are substantial reasons to believe that we are now well into the 'post-truth' era, in which we are to live under conditions in which objective facts and factual rebuttals are found to be much less influential in shaping public opinion in the face of growing power of appeals to emotion and personal belief. At the end of the day the fundamental lesson that one can learn from the dual (and contrasting) role of social media, especially during the pandemic and amidst the super-spread of infodemic, is that reductive, facile and one-sided generalisations about the role of social media are not only fruitless but dangerous.

Democracy, at least in the sense of multiverse of voices, cannot but come under severe strain with the way social media operates, notwithstanding its potential to firm up democracy. A closer look at the modes of functioning of the exceptionally powerful 'platform actors' substantiates the perplexing point. It will be no exaggeration to state that many of our thoughts and actions are now controlled by these platforms. To think that we have autonomy in taking a leaf or two out of media-sourced information and develop our 'own' thinking is to remain completely oblivious to the fact that we are increasingly being made to live in a 'bubble' of communication by the social media overlords. This is precisely the core of the platform politics. One may call it a script or a game or a combination of both, But the crux of the matter is that there is an extremely sophisticated design by social media to subtly enforce 'willing suspension of disbelief' (which incidentally was the prime condition, as per Lewis Carroll, of Alice's entry to the allegorical wonderland). In the social media-sponsored wonderland the users who themselves are nothing but 'products' put up for sale in the advertising market to earn astronomical profit, are not entitled to be thinking beings. It is sometimes pointed out that by favouring the case of social media for the first time in human history importance is being paid to the demand side of the information/communication order, thereby reversing the age-old practice of transactions dictated by the supply side. The statement is apparently true but inherently misleading as it averts unravelling the inner modes of operation of social media. The modes have to be analysed with reference to their unavoidable source in various business models. With persuasive technology and growth strategies/tactics as twin pillars these models indulge in bleeding-edge competition among themselves for profit maximisation.

To move deeper into the process, the highly sophisticated and effective business models are part of the broader phenomenon of 'attention economy', the latest creation of the informational capitalism, which facilitates and in turn is facilitated by social media. Social media is bent on maximising attention of users through engaging them on screen of the gadgets possessed by the users. The engagement time is its driving force, the foundation of its profit maximisation goal. It is important to be aware of the tremendous force with which the users' attention, orientations and the behavioural patterns are monetised to sustain and calibrate the attention economy. The lesser the degree of user autonomy, the greater the potential for profit generation. The earlier perception that the advent of social media would necessarily make the state/government hostile to it has proved to be only partially true. It is because the appropriation of user autonomy in thinking and practice also serves the purpose of those who run the state/government and publicise netizenship at the cost of citizenship. Citizens endowed with critical faculty come in the way of 'friction-free' governing. The rise of 'click'-active netizens, communicating from their respective digital nodes and avoiding 'social distancing', serves the interests of governments and social media, with a strategic mix of political and commercial interests. This is why one would find occasional instances of friction between government and social media giants but a general absence of commitment to create regulatory mechanisms on the part of most governments (excepting the authoritarian ones which do so for illicit transgression on the freedom of expression) to ensure more constructive role for social media. India is a classic example in this regard. Facebook fended off stiff resistance from the TRAI (Telecom Regulatory Authority of India) when it tried to introduce its Free Basics Scheme in India in which a platform for access to select websites for free access by local audiences was sought to be created. Despite Zuckerberg's efforts to convince the apex regulatory agency about the scheme's 'great value' it had to be abandoned on the grounds that it would result in restricting users to certain sites patronised only by Facebook. Facebook India has also faced the allegations about receiving huge funds from both the ruling and the opposition parties before elections. In late October, 2020, the public policy chief of Facebook India resigned following probing questions from a parliamentary committee about certain 'undesirable activities'. There were allegations from the opposition parties like the Indian National Congress that she had continued to favour the dominant ruling party of India in many ways, including showing 'political bias', especially in not deleting the 'inappropriate contents' concerning the minority communities, which were allegedly circulated by the members of the ruling party. Another controversy involving Twitter in India relates to its declaration of itself as a 'platform', rather than a publisher, to evade responsibility for the content posted on its site. The

Parliamentary Committee on Data Privacy Bill raised "strong objection" to such move in January, 2020. These developments indicate the need for some substantive regulatory steps. After a long gap the Government of India introduced certain regulations[3] on social media while acknowledging its role in 'empowering people' and asking it to do business in the country.

To reiterate, AI remains the guiding technology for social media. AI research, as an *Analytics Insight* account by Disha Sinha (2021) describes, opens up an extraordinary combination and simultaneous 'real life' applications of the potential of Deep Machine Learning, Natural Language Processing, Robotics, Speech Expert System, Computer Vision, Artificial Neural Network, Recommender System, Reinforcement Learning, Biometrics and Computational Biology. Social media's astonishingly meticulous and exponential collection of user databases and profiles, propelled by AI, enables it not only to impose surveillance on its users but also to manipulate their identity to 'supply' any amount of specific data on demand by clients with commercial and/or political motives. Its business models, to be referred below, which are foundationally meant to calibrate the attention economy, are intimately connected with its own political ambition to be simultaneously a sponsor and an ally of the ruling forces around the world. The ambitious grabbing of commercial power goes hand in hand with the aspiration to be a part of the political power game. One of the most discussed issues in recent times, highlighting the state-social media entente, has been the alleged involvement of Facebook as a 'collaborator' of Russia in manipulating the American presidential election in 2016, allegedly in denigrating and vilifying the Democrat candidate, Hilary Clinton and in installing Donald Trump to power. (In a twist of events, it is the same Trump whose account Facebook would temporarily suspend after the mob violence in Capitol Hill in January, 2021, on the grounds that the outgoing President's social media messages had instigated the incident). The presidential election is also connected with the infamous case of the Facebook–Cambridge Analytica data breach, revealed in 2018. It was a novel instance of manipulation in which more than 87 million unsuspecting Facebook users' profiles were harvested illegally by Cambridge Analytica, a company specialising in data mining and data analysis. The purpose was to develop a software to predict and influence the choice of the voters. This incident, widely described as a scandal, was only a symptom of the ambitious process of combining business with politics. Incidentally, Hilary Clinton was also made a victim of Russia-sponsored political advertisements which unleashed personal attack on her with the intention of destroying her image. The fact remains that despite having the greater number of popular votes she lost the race by a whisker, with some 'swings' often interpreted as orchestrated. In crass commercial terms it was a classic case of (user) data being sold for gaining astronomical profit, both political and commercial.

The restlessness of social media keeps it going and facilitates its attempt to achieve what till the other day was seemingly impossible. There is relentless systematic and systemic attempt, backed up by finest technologies, to reduce micro-targeted users to the state of 'zombies'. Zombies are individuals with atrophied ability, who exist by remaining unconscious and guided by others, rather than as 'thinking actors' or 'acting thinkers'. This maximises the predictive capacity of the models devised by social media. The fiscal dynamics of social media is always prioritised over everything else. This account of the inner modus operandi of social media may provoke one to contend that in a given situation the ethical concerns reflected in the community guidelines of various social media giants may at best have more intrinsic value and less use value; at worst, it may be an instance just showcasing moral concern. One exceptionally revealing Netflix docudrama, The Social Dilemma, narrates how social media by design literally celebrates addiction, polarisation, radicalisation, outrage-ification and vanity-ification to manipulate user behaviour. The process has also been brought under an umbrella-term, 'Zuckerberg-ification'. One of the most attractive features of the docudrama is that apart from the interviews of academics specialising in the study of social media it is based on extensive interviews of a number of the chief architects of social media algorithm and former top officials of some of the major social media platforms. Facebook has reacted to the contents of the docudrama with a rather unconvincing rebuttal, arguing that its own algorithms are meant to 'create value' and not addiction. It has also borrowed the age-old argument of the mainstream media that advertisements only serve to provide free contents to the audiences. But in any case, Facebook remains 'besieged'. In December, 2020, it faced a severe indictment from the US Federal Trade Commission, which, along with 46 states, filed an anti-trust lawsuit against it. The tech behemoth was accused of abusing its monopoly powers in social networking by taking over rival platforms illegally to 'squelch' competitive threats and ensuring its 'unchecked power' over information and social interactions. The Commission as a solution wanted Facebook to divest Instagram and WhatsApp, a measure if implemented would deal a severe blow not just to WhatsApp and Instagram but also to Facebook's commercial motives and image management. *The New York Times* observes (Kang and Isaac, 2020:1) that if Facebook breaks up it may 'remake the social media industry'. Facebook on the other hand is making efforts to integrate all its subsidiaries, including WhatsApp. In one such major manifestation the 'take it or leave it' Terms of Service of WhatsApp was initiated in some countries, including India, since the beginning of 2021. It required users to agree to the sharing of WhatsApp information with Facebook for 'business purposes', which has lot of implications for data protection and data privacy and data sovereignty. There is little doubt that the monopolistic tendencies of the tech giants are providing stiff challenge to the anti-trust actions; here one can passingly refer to Amazon which is in a different stratosphere in so far as the monopolistic practices are concerned.

No discussion on social media is complete without reference to algorithm landscape. Algorithms are apparently technological issues but nowadays they have been injected with political values. In the domain of computer science it is a set of mathematical rules of calculations and problem-solving instructions for computer-mediated computation with well-defined and sequence-specified actions. In the case of social media its utility value lies in upending social behaviour, in designing programmes to maximise user engagement with gadgets, to the extent of blindly leading them by its dictated contents. Algorithm is the foundational tool with which social media seeks to indulge in 'perfect' prediction of which statement is to be liked or disliked, which one to be shared most among whom and so forth. A number of researchers are now involved in exploring the new and fascinatingly complex relations between algorithms and the shaping of the imaginary and practice of security, and the nature and extent of a possible shift, if not a wholesale paradigm change, in the political rationality of security. A section of such research has specific focus on global health security and the algorithmic security technologies, with special reference to outbreak communication vis-à-vis diseases of such magnitude like HIV/AIDS, SARS, pandemic flu, MERS (Middle East Respiratory Syndrome), Ebola, Zika and the mightiest of them all, coronavirus. It is worth mentioning that a number of such studies (such as, Roberts and Elbe, 2016:1–17) are prepared to go at great length beyond the immediate concern to highlight how the algorithmic governmentality impacts the underlying 'problem, nature and role of knowledge' in contemporary security policy – that too with wider political ramifications. Algorithmic governmentality is also found to be a means of possible a 're-globalization of socio-political governmentality' in which social networking sites and social media play a decisive role. The process is supposed to make a shift from a kind of governmentality implemented on national populations through compiling statistics to a sort of governmentality implemented on citizens-users through big data and algorithms – powered by a GAFAM (Google-Amazon-Facebook-Apple-Microsoft) model. The role of data has become a major reference point in understanding our existence. Couldry and Mejias (2019:xvi) raise an ethical concern in this context in asking whether human beings accept a world in which lives are unceasingly appropriated through data for capitalism. Their prime concern is data colonialism, a global process of extraction which they trace back to the days of earlier mode of colonialism and thereafter industrial capitalism. They explain (p. xix) how intertwining social arrangements and technological infrastructures data appropriate and degrade human life on two counts: by way of surveillance and by way of making human life a direct input to capitalist production. Both are linked to extraction of social resources and profit. In a more empirical vein, analysing big data for governmentality, as part of investigating how particular forms of knowledge production and indices guide development efforts, a study (Flyverboma et al., 2017:35–42) conducts malaria tracking in Kenya and come to the conclusion that what kind of problems are being made visible through big data depends to some degree on how the underlying data is visualised and who is captured in the visualisations. This is partly attributed to the inter-dynamics of the sourcing data and synthesising algorithms.

In the so-called best practices of the algorithm-led world data are not something external to our own selves. It is because 'we are data' (Cheney-Lippold, 2017) or 'we are big data' (Klous and Wielaard, 2016), as the scale and impact of datafication are being interpreted in recent times. In *The Weapons of Math Destruction* (2016) data scientist Cathy O'Neil (2016) is emphatic that thanks to the astounding progress in the world of algorithm-sourced big data and models there is apparently still 'no safe zone' for the 'targeted citizens' who are to bear the consequent damage and injustice.

If this be the case, I may add that tinkering with algorithms is not exactly a viable solution as it does not free us from the dictated process in any constructive way. This is exactly why, O'Neil (2016) observes, the likes of otherwise well-meaning policy counselling – that social media companies can modify algorithms to promote trustworthy content, restrict virality, affix warnings or labels to untruthful content, tightly enforce advertising policies, temporarily suspend accounts or provide links to authoritative sources of information – falls flat. She attributes it to the failure to realise that algorithms are created to serve the monopolistic/oligopolistic commercial interests of social media and not to promote public welfare. She, however, insists that beyond the dominant promotion of logistics, profits and efficiency there still lies the unaddressed question of the 'delivery of transparency' – of disclosing the input data that are being used and the results of their 'targeting' activities. One can again refer to the Facebook – Cambridge Analytica case in this context. O'Neil (2016) also calls the dominant tech giants to be obligated to audits. As she argues in the book, the basic issue with the predictive models managing our lives is that they are to be constructed not just from data but from the 'fundamentally moral' choices we make about which data to pay attention to, and which to leave out. Let me emphasise that there lies precisely the question of democratisation of communication. This also brings back the question – in what form 'community', especially its 'autonomy', exists under the dominant political economy of the Information Age. Not the least, there is also the question how the (netizen) community under prevailing circumstances can be guided and injected with ethical values by the very forces whose own ethical base is under suspect. A great knot in the plot is that it is easier to take actions against the users when the issue concerns nudity, but it is lot more difficult to be as restrictive when it concerns the dissemination of fake information on public health. It is true that Facebook and Twitter have erased President Trump's misleading and erroneous messages underestimating the power and danger of coronavirus, but it is not difficult to associate it with some kind of publicity strategy with the purpose of showcasing the credentials of social media. To what extent and with what regularity such actions are taken against numerous misleading messages by others is anyone's guess.

I shall point out that essentially there are four constraints to achieving 'absolute' control by any particular social media baron or big tech corporation. First, the intrinsic and ever-expanding 'massification' impulse and strategy of the cutting-edge information technology, which do not encourage any specific agency, however powerful, from having monopoly control over all users and over all possible interconnected and cross connected information sources and information flows. Thus, while the World Wide Web has proved to be a thoroughly unequal site, much in contrary to its earlier promise of being the largest ever public commons it is not under the sole control of any single big tech overlord. The bleeding-edge competition for control over the virtual world by the big tech corporations ensures that none gets the exclusive control of things. Even in cases when they may have different objectives and functions (say, those of Facebook and Google) each has too great a stake to let the other have such exclusive propriety. The operational logic of informational capitalism would put such exclusivity issue out. It will also be impossible because the rivals would make use of the anti-trust laws to restrain each other from having absolute leverage. This will be so even if in no small measure they may individually have much reservation about the anti-trust laws. Second, the inability of social media to defy and surpass the state power in all possible respects and exert unrestrained power comes into effect. The Chinese or the North Korean restraining treatment meted out to social media may be cited here along with the rider that it goes too far in repressing the freedom of expression too. But even in democratic countries social media can be controlled to some extent if there is appropriate political will and administrative action. In this context, Tristan Harris (2020:11), a former Google executive and an activist exposing the manipulative motives and mechanisms of social media, asserts that in some European countries, in which the General Data Protection Regulation (GDPR) has been passed, Facebook and other big tech corporations could not but implement all of the provisions, including the provision of content moderation, in their platform. The GDPR is a core regulation on data protection and privacy in the European Union and in the European Economic Area. It is composed of seven key principles: lawfulness, fairness and transparency; purpose limitation; data minimisation; accuracy; storage limitation; integrity and confidentiality (security); and accountability. Harris argues that the same set of data protection can be utilised as precedents by other countries to have a check on social media. However, this brings us back to the question of the state/government-social media nexus which serves the interests of both at the direct cost of public interest. Third, there is lack of substantive credibility of big tech corporations themselves to legitimately impose ethical standards on others. The frequent accusations of breaching the anti-trust laws, which most often involve Facebook, Google and Microsoft, is too well-known. The façade of the freedom of expression, constructed by such corporations to defend their actions, does not hold much ground. Here again, Harris (2020:11) raises a pertinent question distinguishing between the freedom of speech and the freedom to reach: 'We can have a right to say something to other people but do we have a God-given right to broadcast to millions of people without accountability?' It is true that when the mainstream media is subject to various regulations the social media remains free from them. Fourth, there is the insurmountable challenge caused by simultaneity of two contradictory acts of social media: the imposition of restrictions on users beyond a limit on the one hand, and self-publicity of being a facilitator of the freedom of expression, on the other hand.

Let me now explain the predicament of social media by referring to two events involving the most powerful social media baron of this era. It is of much significance that while in the aftermath of the US presidential election in 2016 Zuckerberg had aggressively denied any wrongdoing on the part of Facebook and had dismissed the allegation that his organisation had contributed to Trump's win, in his testimony to the European Parliament on 22 May, 2018, he expressed regret that 'mistakes' had been made. He referred to the prevalence of fake news and the practice of developers themselves misusing people's information, further admitting that 'we didn't take a broad enough view of our responsibilities'. Zuckerberg in this context had also suggested that the problems could be fixed through new technology and an investment in extra staff, significantly without making any new pledges for any radical change in Facebook's modus operandi. There lies the catch: the new technology has no compulsion to fix things up against corporate business interest because the two are intimately linked. Nor can a motley group of technologists, who are basically employees, have any power at their disposal to be the sole agents of transformation. What remained unsaid in the whole issue is that even if one hypothetically assumes that good sense would prevail among the social media barons, it itself implies being a bit too optimistic. The fact is that there can be no totally fool-proof mechanism to prevent mis/disinformation because of the compelling expansion of digital technology and its constitutive logic, both in terms of intent and techno-architecture, to facilitate multiple information sources and flows within an overarching order run by informational capitalism.

The search for alternatives goes on in different tone and tenor. In an attempt at in-situ understanding of the power politics of algorithmic life with the specific focus on the material-discursive dimensions of software Bucher (2018) seeks to find a way out in exploring the central question (p. 159) – who or what gets to be part of whatever is being articulated as the algorithm. She studies Google's search algorithms, Facebook's News Feed algorithms and Netflix's collaborative filtering algorithms to scrutinise big data and the immersive capacity based on sociality and connectivity. She pleads for a developed understanding of the mechanics of algorithm rather than treating it as 'black box'. In a more radical vein and in offering greater resistance to algorithm life, Couldry and Mejias plead (2019:111) for a decolonial approach to data to facilitate framing *counter-presents*, the 'alternative understandings of current social realities that allow us to see ourselves as more than mere inputs for capitalism'. They have an ambitious plan of exploring methods for denaturalising the logic of data, critiquing data colonialism, to reimagine different forms of social and economic relations and connections outside of western notions of modernity and western form of reason. Creating counterpresents, according to them, implies several tasks:

i) Engaging in media practices that question how notions of 'progress', 'civilisation', or 'innovation' are equated with data relations as conceptualised by corporate interests.
ii) Reclaiming the agency of the colonised data subject.
iii) Allowing the subjects of data colonialism to imagine a different worldview in which they can locate themselves as fully autonomous actors, beyond data's 'horizon of totality' and with a fully recognised right to challenge the progress of data colonialism.

Such an ambitious project is sought to be undertaken urgently because they argue that data colonialism is in a period of transition, and that an emerging order is yet to come. However, it seems that while such utopian vision is important in itself to visualise an alternative world order, the very order they describe as 'emerging' has already emerged and it has become strong enough to considerably complicate the vision of an alternative order. But arriving at a viable alternative order may not be easy. As long as it is not achieved there is little possibility of any radical transformation of the existing order as mis/disinformation is treated as affordable natural and spontaneous aberrations, not posing any kind of unnerving threat to the order itself. This is why the dominant political economy of the Information Age, mentioned earlier in the discussion, is of great importance. The most enviable thing about capitalism, especially when compared to its contending forces, is its strategic indulgence to the instances of aberrations as long as they remain 'unthreatening' to its basic terms and conditions. With the digital technology emerging as a major propelling force of the informational capitalism there is little possibility of any intrinsic democratic change in the overall plot by those who benefit most out of it. The efforts to expose and change its modus operandi have to come externally, based on the conviction that absolute and total control of our life by new technology is not attainable. This is a point which the critics of informational capitalism have to keep in mind when on occasions they advocate a world free from the suffocating control of digital technology. The conviction on the part of the critics has to continually assert the fact that however meticulous the big corporate forces are in managing the big data the existing physical world is too vast, too dynamic and too diverse to be subject to total control with cent per cent certainty and predictions. In the mind game constructed by informational capitalism and its transgressive technology at this point in time what is of great importance is not to collectively fall prey to a designed belief system which among other things transmits the invincibility of social media and its data power.

Concluding remarks

Without further ado let us accept the fact that infodemic is here to stay. It is because countering it effectively not only involves a sustained struggle against the prevailing information ecosystem but also a decisive struggle against the discriminatory word order. Yet there are possible ways to negotiate with it. Infodemic disturbs the shaping of the information ecosystem by challenging the classical tenets of ideal communication – reliability, credibility, trust and relevance – but as has been pointed out above even those dominant forces contributing to such imbalance for own commercial, economic or political interests cannot have total control over information flows. Here too, the concerned analysts, who look for ways and means of preserving the sanctity of the public sphere as the scaffolding of democratic polity, also have to explore a delicate balance. It is in the sense that on the one hand they have to guard against romanticising 'people' as the repository of freedom of expression and as unwavering agents of inclusive communication, on the other hand they have to resist elitist motives of restraining the freedom of expression. The pandemic situation has already revealed enough to be aware of such a hard but essential task.

Notes

1 In some cases, a subtle distinction is made between 'misinformation' and 'disinformation', though the two terms are closely connected, conceptually and otherwise, and are often used synonymously. Both refer to fake or inaccurate information but a key distinction between them lies in the intention. If it is deliberately created to deceive it has the chance to fall into the category of misinformation. Disinformation generally refers to the intentional cases of creation and dissemination of information. In this chapter, both are given their due importance as major constituents of infodemic and they are being represented as 'mis/disinformation', except in direct quotes and on occasions requiring specific connotations.

2 The close connection between social networking and social media often leads to the use of the two terms interchangeably. Here however, social media is treated as a point of convergence of various sites, online networks and web applications, with heavy user-centric interactive traffic of messages, data, information, ideas and images. The book largely adheres to the view (Meikle, 2016: x) of social media as a particular set/s of technological affordances, of business models and corporate practices, of organisations, and of cultural habits, practices and expectations. In this view 'social media' connotes a specific set of Internet-based, networked communication platforms resting on business models of database, enabling the convergence of public and personal communication. It is a constituent of Government 2.0/Governance 2.0, supposedly characterised by greater citizen access, interaction and participation in policymaking.

3 The key provisions in the guidelines on social media regulation by the Ministry of Information and Broadcasting, Government of India:

- The platforms will have to employ a chief compliance officer, a nodal contact person and a resident grievance officer.
- The self-regulatory body will be headed by a retired judge of the Supreme Court or of a high court, or by a person of eminence from the relevant field, who can issue advisories to the publisher.
- Social media platforms upon being asked either by a court order or a government authority will be required to disclose the first originator of mischievous tweet or message as the case may be. This should be only in relation to sovereignty and integrity of India, security of the state, public order, relations with foreign states, or rape, sexually explicit content and the likes.
- All social media platforms will have two categories of intermediaries. The central government is to notify the number of users for a significant social media intermediary. The intermediaries must have a grievance redressal mechanism. They will also have to name a grievance officer who shall register the grievance within twenty four hours and ensure disposal in 15 days. The intermediary will publish a monthly compliance report mentioning the details of complaints received and action taken on the complaints as well as details of contents removed proactively.
- The person appointed as chief compliance officer shall be a resident of India. He/she will be responsible for ensuring compliance with rules and acts. The nodal contact person will be responsible for 24×7 coordination with law enforcement agencies. The resident grievance officer shall perform all functions under grievance redressal mechanism. All intermediaries shall have a physical contact address in India published on website or mobile app or both.
- To ensure online safety and dignity of users, especially women users, intermediaries have been asked to remove or disable access within twenty four hours of receipt of complaints of contents that exposes the private areas of individuals, show such

individuals in full or partial nudity or in sexual act or is in the nature of impersonation including morphed images.

- Self-classification of contents into five age-based categories: U (Universal), U/A 7+, U/A 13+, U/A 16+, and A (Adult). Platforms will be required to implement parental locks for content classified as U/A 13+ or higher, and reliable age verification mechanisms for content classified as 'A'.
- Voluntary verification mechanism of users: all social media platforms will have a provision for voluntary verification mechanism of the users. If the platforms seek to disable access to the content of any social media user they are required to give reasons and also hear the concerned party out.

Source: https://timesofindia.indiatimes.com/business/india-business/government-guidelines-on-social-media-regulation-key-points/articleshow/81207213.cms. Accessed 30 March, 2021.

CONCLUSION

Future tense

What does the COVID-19 virus leave us with? One possible and somewhat uncomfortable response to the question might be that it leaves us with the virus itself. In essence the implication is that even if it physically leaves us, it will not go away from our life any time soon. The second wave of the pandemic, which made its presence felt since December, 2020, has proved to be more infectious than the first. The third strain followed by raising its head here and there, initially in Russia, China and UK. Vaccines are being discovered and administered from multiple sources but scepticism and anxiety remain abound. 'The worst is yet to come' and 'Corona is our future', two familiar *new normal* sayings warn. There is at times a thin line between speculation and prediction. Whether the virus will ever physically leave us is also a tricky question because biologists, virologists and epidemiologists have warned that its multiple mutations are natural. Thus there is no surprise in it having successive strains and having its continuity in manifest and latent forms. Such process will be part of the 'next normal'. Even if we hypothetically assume that it will leave us, never to show its face again, we have to live with its devastating consequences for a long time. The deadly virus may have operated with a specific lifespan in human body and its manifestations and consequences may have taken place within a particular span of time but there is no doubt that its impact will remain for decades.

The pandemic created by COVID-19 virus is certainly not the first one in history. Even in the corona category of viruses it is not the first but only the seventh in line of succession. But as has been asserted by many around, and also quite a few times in our discussion, it has displayed unparalleled spread, depth and astonishing range not only in medical, biological, virological, epidemiological and other health fields but also in geopolitical, economic, political, social, psychological and cultural arenas. It has changed the world around us in just few days, which otherwise would have taken not just years but multiple decades to occur. Moving paradoxically, it has on the one hand shown 'equality' in physically infecting people irrespective of

DOI: 10.4324/9781003247388-7

race, ethnicity, social strata, economic conditions, ideological and political affiliations and religious attachments. On the other hand, it has aggravated inequality and severe discrimination in terms of access to treatment, loss of lives and livelihood, hunger, starvation, creation of panic, anxiety, paranoia and so forth, putting underprivileged and marginalised people in extreme conditions, threatening their life and very survival. There is no other option but to visualise our future in this backdrop. Before making some general observations based on few key points which have been expanded in the book let me reaffirm what many a time has been mentioned earlier— that the only certainty about the pandemic is its uncertainty. The contention, which does not sound pleasant to the ears, may briefly be explained here for the last time.

It is by now evident that there could be three possible ways of negotiating and countering the pandemic globally. First, to impose strict lockdown, quarantine and social distancing norms and initiate mass testing and vaccination for a long time to detach the chains of infection. Australia, for example, found much success in having a four month-long lockdown since July, 2020. Some countries, it has been noted, have successfully followed the measures mainly because of the 'conformist' population. However, it has been impossible to follow such restrictive practices in all the countries of the world for a variety of reasons. It is not just because of economic, social and cultural factors but also because many political leaders became excessively confident and took the pandemic too lightly, deliberately underestimating the advice of specialists and social activists. Second, the herd immunity is often publicised as the faster way of countering COVID-19 but the fact remains that leaving a substantial section of population dependent on another section to develop immunity in 'course of time' puts too many people at risk. It is particularly risky in populous countries which run greater risks of 'community transmission' of infection. Third, the zoning approach, which calls for more intense quarantine measures in the 'red zones', that is the areas most infected, and leaves the 'yellow zones', that is the least affected areas undisturbed, is also problematic. It is especially so in societies where self-discipline is not a strong social trait. This leaves us with no consensual way of negotiating the virus and the pandemic. The uncertainty is even more compounded by the fact that there is no firm epidemiological guarantee about the seasonality of the virus, its changing modes of adaptation as seasons change. Even if vaccines continue to be invented, they need to go through regular rigorous testing and they have to be distributed in exceptionally huge quantity around the world. Moreover, it will take a long time to measure their efficacy in the form of duration of immunity among vaccinated population. In the 73rd World Health Assembly virtual meet on 18–19 May, 2020, the WHO has affirmed that health is the foundation of social, economic and political stability. But at the same time it issued a warning note that we must make preparations for the next pandemic on the basis of 'science, solutions and solidarity'. Yet, as experience shows, there are too many constraints at work.

To describe the future as tense is not to press the panic button harder. Nor is it to be a cynical naysayer. It is more of an effort to come out of the anthropocentric conceit that much concerns the 'end of the pandemic' idea. It is more of an outcome of the hard realisation that it is not just a question of decline in the rate of economic growth or that of slowing down of societies but also in much impactful way it is a question of the 'modern' civilisation itself having faltered. The 'normal' of the pre-corona times can never be resumed, at least not in the exact form. But the past remains a lesson to learn from the present crisis and plan the future. To qualify the point further, the future lying ahead may be categorised into 'proximate' and 'distant'. Insofar as the proximate future is concerned the post-pandemic scene is bound to be marked by an uphill struggle on all possible fronts to reorganise life and reframe or reformulate many of our hitherto treasured ideas, practices and beliefs.

To what extent we can do it will determine the nature of the distant future as there is a clear linkage between the two different temporal phases, 'near' and 'long'. The first one is the key to determining the other one which is more distant but bound to come closer with each passing day. The pandemic, as the book reveals and asserts, has made things complicated by exposing a huge number of fault lines and even aggravating many. To what extent the tension will have its imprint in our future will depend on the degree to which we are ready negotiate the known-unknown dialectics. Such dialectics, as it is explained at the very early part of the book, involves the multidimensional process of *knowing the unknown* and *unknowing the known*. Notably, a section of the ongoing debate on the pandemic still concerns the question whether it was 'plandemic', a planned event by some key corporate giants from as different domains as high tech and pharmaceuticals, in league with some powerful states to take greater control of the global political economy. Such logic proves that there is lack of definite knowledge even about the 'core' status of the crisis. One can venture to add that the process of coming to terms with the pandemic also involves *knowing the known again*. The entrenched complexity is a motif of what has been described in the book as the flexi-modern times. There is not much doubt that the 'creative tension' in this process is sure to contribute in its own way to the making of the post-pandemic future, if there is any.

That the future is bound to be made tense by the act of governing is much evident from the discussion in the book, which depicts how the intersection and interplay of state/government and the market/corporate forces make the search for solutions to many issues of public concern not just complicated but elusive. The pandemic has indeed made the 'shadowy' areas of governing more transparent by showing that not just health policies but public policies in general are not to be mechanically and technocratically associated with welfarist, solution-oriented motives. Strategic inaction and/or ingrained deficiency make their latent presence in 'good governance'. On occasions, when threatened or directly confronted with decisive challenges expose their incompetence and callousness the rulers strike back with inherently false people-centric rhetoric, histrionics and more penetratingly, with bio-political actions seeking to colonise critical faculty of citizens by favouring 'herd instinct' as the way of automated social control. In a broader way it exposes the danger of technological micro-management of individual behaviours to enforce public discipline, not just during the pandemic times but also otherwise. The regimentation dream of banishing dissent by asserting the material immortality of technology is very much on and on a number of occasions it becomes the reality. However, such effort cannot achieve the level it aspires to attain simply because very often the wide variations in human nature evoke very different interpretations and responses to the identical actions and strategies. As has been noted, this is where and how politics in the constructive sense of the term survives and makes its presence felt.

The book also reveals that human communication which, especially with the incredible advance of digital technology had already broken new grounds and reached new heights, made further twists and turns in the pandemic times. It apparently became more intensely used medium for common people during the lockdowns and the quarantine days. But in more extensive and vigorous ways it also became a bridge-building force between governments and corporates along with social media seeking to consolidate its position with more penetrating but less ambiguous strategisation. In the whole affair, when crisis times demanded more transparent, credible and reliable information it became all the more clear that false and fake data and information would circulate more than ever before. As has been noted, one of the most striking developments in the millennial communication order is the pro-active role of ordinary people in creating and circulating fake and false information. It also involves developing toxic and vitriolic social discourses by taking advantage of the pandemic situation, lack of conclusive scientific evidence about the virus and large-scale uncertainty, insecurity and gloom all around. In this specific context the pandemic has certainly contributed to greater awareness of the need to pay for more attention to the conditions of the ordinary people but at the same time it has also made social analysts all the more conscious of the problem of utopian thinking about the 'public sphere' based on free and fair communication among and by people. Overall, the pandemic has shown sufficient capacity to create disorder of the first category on various fronts but with the infodemic let loose, as we have seen, it also leaves its indelible mark insofar as the communication order is concerned.

Bringing some order into the disorder requires a collective resistance in a deeper political sense – beyond some tactical and strategic manoeuvring here and there. As there is no geometric blueprint to fall back on, in more subjective terms the fight against the pandemic and the efforts to ensure a safer and more secure future involve enhancement of solidarity. Solidarity in turn depends on reducing mutual hostility and antagonism to a considerable extent at multiple levels. This reduction process invariably encompasses the local, regional, international and global arenas in a single spectrum. The biological way of countering the pandemic may need the development of 'herd immunity' but in social terms in a world that is still torn with relational cracks and fissures the 'herd instinct' which generates a resolve to fight the crisis on the basis of 'we feeling' is very weak and the (mutual) trust level is abysmally low. There is a difference between 'being in the world' and 'being of the world' and the blame game on various fronts goes on. The fact that the pandemic is not just a health crisis but an existential crisis engulfing all spheres of life has resulted in intense competition among all. The granular competition is there at the individual level as the economy is hard hit and the social fabric is under severe strain with anxiety, panic and mutual suspicion riding high. One could not find impressive cooperative performance of countries in treatment protocols and therapeutics. At a later stage and at another level there is even an unhealthy competition among nations with regard to the 'first access' to the vaccine. The term 'coronationalism' marked by closed borders and obsessive protectionism, is followed by 'vaccine nationalism'. There are calls for the elimination of patents of the vaccines, but it will not be easy to implement in a world in which 'it's our own' kind of national sentiment is mixed up with steep profit motive of the pharmaceutical behemoths. At its foundation it involves the tricky issue of intellectual property rights (IPR). The global economy being under severe strain and the conductors of governance looking for a fig leaf to hide their failure the scenario is even more complicated than is thought of in the first instance. The global governance thesis, including the global health governance regime, is facing extreme strains with the growing atomisation of the international order caused among other factors by the weakening spirit of multilateralism. It is a settled scientific fact that there is a strong connection between the nature of the climate and the possibility of having pandemics in the planet. Then again, the abject failure, even while facing the scare of coronavirus pandemic, to reach any kind of consensus regarding the climate change issue, only proves the difficulty of reaching minimal consensus on vital issues. Under such circumstances any hasty or hold-all kind of solution with an absolute principle at its base would only be self-defeating, especially if one considers the fact that no two countries are perfectly at ease with each other or for that matter no two societies are ever fully the same.

One only wishes one could have a more optimistic and reassuring tone and tenor in the concluding observations here. But let me iterate that if there is any lack of definitive and optimistic observations about the post-pandemic future it is a natural consequence of the fact that we are yet to decide how to reset ourselves to give a fitting reply to the pandemic itself and to adjust to the complex and volatile environment created by it. This is despite the fact that COVID-19 in certain ways has proved to be a boon in disguise. In a world which has long been habituated to talking without speaking and hearing without listening it has provided an opportunity to rethink our ideas and lifestyle in deeper ways and thus reorient the dominant narrative of development. The issues are not just changing dining habits, partying, work styles and so forth. Nor are they only about scaling up new technology, and strategic-tactical tinkering with business models and public policies. Deep down it concerns cultural practice of a different kind. It involves a steady 'supply chain' of humanism and humanitarian motives and actions. It is fundamentally about changing values, ethics and mindsets – of replacing atomisation of self and social recession. One can see lot of trend analyses being done, many sophisticated simulated models being constructed and fast-track publications coming out and making confident claims and 'reliable' and 'accurate' predictions about the post-corona future. But being too segmental they lose the sight of the woods by only counting the trees. When it comes to visualising the future in terms of pandemic (or epidemic) preparedness much depends on how we learn from the past and negotiate the present. The COVID-19 pandemic having proved to be a civilisational crisis it is better to sign off, as is being done here, with a tantalisingly open stance.

BIBLIOGRAPHY

Accessnow Report. 2020. 'Fighting Misinformation and Defending Free Expression during COVID-19: Recommendations for States accessnow.org', https://www.accessnow.org/cms/assets/uploads/2020/04/Fighting-misinformation-and-defending-free-expression-during-COVID-19-recommendations-for-states-1.pdf Accessed 21 September, 2020.

Achcar, Gilbert. 2020. 'Covid-19 Pandemic and Afterwards? Self-Extinction of Neoliberalism? Don't Bet on It', *Europe Solidaire Sans Frontières*, 24 April, http://www.europe-solidaire.org/spip.php?article53164 Accessed 10 August, 2020.

Adams, Rachel. 2017. 'Michel Foucault: 'Biopolitics and Biopower'', *Critical Legal Thinking*, 10 May, https://criticallegalthinking.com/2017/05/10/michel-foucault-biopolitics-biopower/ Accessed 19 November. 2020.

Agamben, Giorgio, 2005. *State of Exception*, Translated by K. Attell. Chicago: University of Chicago Press.

Agamben, Giorgio. 2020a. '*L'invenzione di un'epidemia', Quodlibet*, 26 February. www.quodlibet.it/giorgio-agamben-l-invenzione-di-un-epidemia. I have used the English version, 'Coronavirus and Philosophers: Giorgio Agamben--- The Invention of an Epidemic', *European Journal of Psychoanalysis*, www.journal-psychoanalysis.eu/coronavirus-and-philosophers/ Accessed 1 July, 2020.

Agamben, Giorgio. 2020b. 'Contagion', https://enoughisenough14.org/2020/03/20/giorgio-agamben-contagion/ Accessed 3 August, 2020.

Agamben, Giorgio. 2021. 'On the Government of the Faceless and the Deathless', *Autonomies*, 4 May, https://autonomies.org/2021/05/giorgio-agamben-on-the-government-of-the-faceless-and-the-deathless/ Accessed 19 May, 2021.

Aiyar, Pallavi. 2020. 'COVID-19: The Ideology-Agnostic Contagion', *Mathrubhumi* (English Edition), 10 April, https://english.mathrubhumi.com/features/specials/covid-19-the-ideology-agnostic-contagion-1.4680331 Accessed 14 July, 2020.

al-Basam, Darim. 2020. 'The Coronavirus: Sociology of a Pandemic', *The Gulf Times*, 2 May. www.gulf-times.com/story/662204/Sociology-of-the-pandemic Accessed 15 May, 2020.

Alles, Michael. 2009. 'Editorial: Governance in the Age of Unknown Unknowns', *International Journal of Disclosure and Governance*, 6, 85–88.

Anderson, Janna and Lee Rainie. 2017. 'The Future of Truth and Misinformation Online', Place not mentioned: Pew Research Centre-Elon University, 1–90.

Article 1. 2020. 'Viral Lies: Misinformation and the Coronavirus', *Policy Brief*, London: Article 19 – Free Word Centre, 1–21.

Bang, Henrik P. 2003. *Governance as Social and Political Communication*, Manchester and New York: Manchester University Press.

Barrelet, Clara, Mathilde Bourrier, Claudine Burton-Jeangros and Melinee Schindler. 2013. 'Unresolved Issues in Risk Communication Research: the Case of the H1N1 Pandemic (2009–2011)', *Influenza and Other Respiratory Viruses* 7 (Suppl. 2), 114–119.

Bauman, Zygmunt. 1991. *Modernity and Ambivalence*, Cambridge, MA: Polity Press.

Bauman, Zygmunt. 1997. *Postmodernity and Its Discontents*, Cambridge: Polity.

Bauman, Zygman. 2000. *Liquid Modernity*. Cambridge, MA: Polity Press.

Bauman, Zygmunt. 2011. *Culture in a Liquid Modern World*, Cambridge, MA: Polity Press.

Beck, Ulrich. 1992. *Risk Society: Towards a New Modernity*, Thousand Oaks, CA: Sage.

Beck, Ulrich. 1997. *The Reinvention of Politics: Rethinking Modernity in the Global Social Order*, Cambridge: Polity Press.

Bell, Daniel. 1960. *The End of Ideology: On the Exhaustion of Political Ideas in the Fifties*, New York: Free Press.

Bell, Stephen and Andrew Hindmoor. 2009. *Rethinking Governance: The Centrality of the State in Modern Society*, Cambridge: Cambridge University Press.

Best, Steven and Douglas Kellner. 1991. *Postmodern Theory: Critical Interrogations*, London: Macmillan.

Bevir, Mark. 2010. *Democratic Governance*, New Jersey: Princeton University Press.

Bevir, Mark and R. A. W. Rhodes. 2011. 'The Stateless State', in Mark Bevir ed., *The Sage Handbook of Governance*, London: Sage Publications, 203–217.

Brennen, J. Scott, Felix M. Simon, Philip N. Howard and Rasmus Kleis Nielsen. 2020. *Types, Sources, and Claims of COVID-19 Misinformation*, Oxford: Reuters Institute-University of Oxford, https://reutersinstitute.politics.ox.ac.uk/types-sources-and-claims-covid-19-misinformation Accessed 23 September, 2020.

Briggs, Charles L. and Daniel C. Hallin. 2007. 'Biocommunicability: The Neoliberal Subject and Its Contradictions in News Coverage of Health Issues', *Social Text 93*, 25(4), 43–66.

Bucher, Taina. 2018. *If... Then Algorithmic Power and Politics*, New York: Oxford University Press.

Burchell, Graham, Colin Gordon and Peter Miller eds. 1991. *The Foucault Effect: Studies in Governmentality*, Chicago, IL University of Chicago Press.

Cahoone, Lawrence E. 1996. *From Modernism to Postmodernism: An Anthology*, Cambridge, MA: Blackwell Publishers.

Caliskan, Koray and Donald MacKenzie. 2020. 'Of Viruses and Men: The Dangerous Pandemic in the Social Sciences', 15 April,www.eurozine.com/of-viruses-and-men/ Accessed 15 April, 2020.

Camus, Albert. 2010 [1946]. *The Plague*, London: Penguin.

Carney, Terry and Belinda Bennett. 2014. 'Framing Pandemic Management: New Governance, Science or Culture?' *Health Sociology Review*, 23(2), 136–147.

Carter, Nick. 2020. 'The Neil Ferguson Affair Shows the Limits of Science During COVID-19', *Coindesk*, 4 June. www.coindesk.com/the-neil-ferguson-affair-shows-the-limits-of-science-during-covid-19 Accessed 4 July.

Castel, Robert. 1991. 'From Dangerousness to Risk', in Graham Burchell, Colin Gordon and Peter Miller eds., *The Foucault Effect: Studies in Governmentality*, Chicago, IL: University of Chicago Press, 281–298.

CDC (Centers for Disease Control and Prevention). 1997. *Principles of Community Engagement*, Atlanta, GA: CDC/ATSDR Committee on Community Engagement.

Cereceda, Rafael. 2020a. 'What We know and Don't Know about the COVID-19 Coronavirus', *Euronews*, 27 March. www.euronews.com Accessed 3 July.

Cereceda, Rafael. 2020b. 'New Coronavirus Not the Real Killer: It's the Patient's Immune System Damaging Vital Organs', *Euronews*, 9 April. www.euronews.com Accessed 3 July.

Chambers, Simone. 2020. 'Truth, Deliberative Democracy, and the Virtues of Accuracy: Is Fake News Destroying the Public Sphere?' *Political Studies*, 1–17. https://journals.sagepub.com/doi/full/10.1177/0032321719890811 Accessed 7 October, 2020.

Chandran, Rina. 2020. 'ANALYSIS-Privacy Concerns as India Pushes Digital Health Plan, IDs', *Thompson Reuters Foundation*, 22 September, https://www.reuters.com/article/india-health-tech-idUKL8N2G536U Accessed 19 May, 2021.

Chater, Nick. 2020. 'Facing Up to the Uncertainties of COVID-19', *Nature Human Behaviour*, 4, 439, 27 March, www.nature.com/articles/s41562-020-0865-2 Accessed 26 June, 2020.

Cheney-Lippold. John. 2017. *We Are Data: Algorithms and the Making of Our Digital Selves*, New York: New York University Press.

Christaens, Tim. 2020. 'Must Society be Defended from Agamben?' *Critical Legal Thinking*, 26 march, https://criticallegalthinking.com/2020/03/26/must-society-be-defended-from-agamben/ Accessed 18 April, 2020.

Cissé, Daouda. 2020. 'COVID-19: Are Scientists Trapped under Policymakers' Poor Leadership?' *global-e*, 13(49), www.21global.ucsb.edu/global-e/july-2020/covid-19-are-scientists-trapped-under-policymakers-poor-leadership Accessed 29 July, 2020.

Cleden, David. 2009. *Managing Project Uncertainty*, Surrey: Gower.

Coombs, W. Timothy. 2009. 'Conceptualizing Crisis Communication', in Robert L. Heath and H. Dan O'Hair eds., *Handbook of Risk and Crisis Communication*, New York and Oxford: Routledge, 99–118.

Corrêa, Sonia. 2020. *Biopolitics & The COVID-19 Pandemic: Feminist Perspectives*, Suva: DAWN (Development Alternatives with Women for a New Era).

Couldry, Nick and Ulises A. Mejias. 2019. *The Costs of Connection: How Data is Colonizing Human Life and Appropriating It for Capitalism*, Stanford, CA: Stanford University Press.

Crouch, Colin. 2016. *The Knowledge Corrupters: Hidden Consequences of the Financial Takeover of Public Life*, Cambridge and Malden: Polity Press.

Crouch, Colin. 2011. *The Strange Non-Death of Neoliberalism*, Cambridge: Polity Press.

Cyranoski, David. 2020. 'The Biggest Mystery: What Will it Take to Trace the Coronavirus Source', *Nature*, 5 June. https://www.nature.com/articles/d41586-020-01541-z Accessed 7 July, 2020.

Dahl, Robert. 1961. *Who Governs? Democracy and Power in an American City*, New Haven: Yale University Press.

Data Sheet I. 2020. 'Global Social Media Overview', https://datareportal.com/social-media-users Accessed 28 September, 2020.

Data Sheet II. 2020. 'Social Media Statistics 2020: Top Networks by the Numbers', https://dustinstout.com/social-media-statistics/ Accessed 28 September, 2020.

Davis, Mark and Davina Lohm. 2020. *Pandemics, Publics, and Narrative*, New York: Oxford University Press.

Das Gupta, Debasree and David W. S. Wong. 2020. 'No More "Social Distancing" but Practice Physical Separation', *Canadian Journal of Public Health*, 111(4), 488–489.

Degerman, Dan, Matthew Flinders and Matthew Thomas Johnson. 2020. 'In Defence of Fear: COVID-19, Crises and Democracy', *Critical Review of International Social and Political Philosophy*, 1–22. https://www.tandfonline.com/doi/pdf/10.1080/13698230.2020.1834744?needAccess=true Accessed 19 April, 2021.

DELWP. 2015. *An introduction to Engagement. Effective Engagement: Building Relationships with Community and Other Stakeholders*. Book 1, Department of Environment, Land, Water and Planning, Melbourne: State Government of Victoria, 1–35.

Dempsey, Sarah E. 2010. 'Critiquing Community Engagement', *Management Communication Quarterly* 24(3), 359–390.

Desikan, Anita, Taryn MacKinney and Gretchen Goldman. 2020. 'Let the Scientists Speak How CDC Experts Have Been Sidelined during the COVID-19 Pandemic', *Union of Concerned Scientists*, 1–5. https://www.ucsusa.org/sites/default/files/2020-05/let-the-scientists-speak.pdf Accessed 8 April, 2021.

Deutsch, Karl W. 1963. *The Nerves of Government: Models of Political Communication and Control*, New York: The Free Press of Glencoe.

Dijck, José van, Thomas Poell and Martijn de Waal. 2018. *The Platform Society: Public Values in a Connective World*, New York: Oxford University Press.

Dingwall, Robert, Lily M Hoffman and Karen Staniland. 2013. 'Introduction: Why a *Sociology* of Pandemics?' *Sociology of Health and Illness*, 35(2), 167–173.

Doerr, Neriko Musha. 2009. 'Introduction: Knowledge, Ignorance, and Relations of Dominance', *Critical Studies in Education*, 50(3), 289–294.

Dryzek, John. S. 2007. 'Networks and Democratic Ideals: Equality, Freedom, and Communication', in Eva Sørensen and Jacob Torfing eds., *Theories of Democratic Network Governance*, Hampshire: Palgrave Macmillan, 262–273.

Dryzek, John S. and Simon Niemeyer. 2008. 'Discursive Representation', *American Political Science Review*, 102(4), 481–493.

Edkins, Jenny. 2008. 'Biopolitics, Communication and Global Governance', *Review of International Studies*, 34, 211–232.

Epstein, Steven. 1996. *Impure Science: AIDS, Activism, and the Politics of Knowledge*, Berkley: University of California Press.

Epstein, Steven. 2020. 'COVID-19 and the Politics of Knowledge (Science, Knowledge, and Technology)', *Footnotes*, 48(3), May–June. https://www.asanet.org/news-events/footnotes/may-jun-2020/research-policy/covid-19-and-politics-knowledge-science-knowledge-and-technology Accessed 1 July, 2020.

Fazi, Thomas. 2020. 'Could COVID-19 Vanquish Neoliberalism?' *Unherd*, 6 April, https://unherd.com/2020/04/could-covid-19-vanquish-neoliberalism/ Accessed 1 May, 2020.

Ferrar, Jeremy. 2020. ''Forget Any False Sense of Security: We Are Still at the Start of the Global Pandemic', *The Guardian*, 2 July. https://www.theguardian.com/commentisfree/2020/jul/02/security-global-pandemic-vaccines-treatments-coronavirus Accessed 3 July.

Flyverboma, Mikkel, Anders Koed Madsenb and Andreas Rasche. 2017. 'Big data as Governmentality in International Development: Digital Traces, Algorithms, and Altered Visibilities'. *The Information Society*, 33:1, 35–42.

Foster, John Bellamy and Intan Suwandi. 2020. 'COVID-19 and Catastrophe Capitalism: Commodity Chains and Ecological-Epidemiological-Economic Crises', *Monthly Review*, 72(2), 1 June, https://monthlyreview.org/2020/06/01/covid-19-and-catastrophe-capitalism/ Accessed 8 June, 2020.

Foucault, Michel. 1990. *The History of Sexuality, Volume 1: An Introduction*, Translated by Robert Hurley, New York: Vintage.

Foucault, Michel. 1991. 'Governmentality', in Graham Burchell, Colin Gordon and Peter Miller eds., *The Foucault Effect: Studies in Governmentality*, Chicago, IL: University of Chicago Press, 87–104.

Foucault, Michel. 1995. *Discipline and Punish: The Birth of the Prison*, Translated by Alan Sheridan, New York: Vintage.

Foucault, Michel. 2006. *History of Madness*, ed. Jean Khalfa, Translated by Jonathan Murphy, London and New York: Routledge.

Foucault, Michel. 2013 [1976]. 'Society Must be Defended: Lecture at the College de France, March 17, 1976', in Timothy Campbell and Adam Sitze eds. *Biopolitics: A Reader*, Durham: Duke University Press, 61–81.

French, Martin and Torin Monahan. 2020. 'Dis-ease Surveillance: How Might Surveillance Studies Address COVID-19?' *Surveillance & Society*, 18(1), 1–11.

Friedman, Thomas L. 2000. *The Lexus and the Olive Tree: Understanding Globalization*, New York: Anchor Books.

Ghosal, Somak. 2020. 'Open Book?' *Index on Censorship*, 41(2), 53–55.

Ghosh, Sujay. 2021. 'India and the Pandemic: Democratic Governance at Crossroads', *International Journal of Asian Studies*, 1–20, https://doi.org/10.1017/S1479591421000188 Accessed 17 May, 2021.

Giddens, Anthony. 1990. *The Consequences of Modernity*, Stanford, CA: Stanford University Press.

Giroux, Henry A. 2020. 'The COVID-19 Pandemic Is Exposing the Plague of Neoliberalism', *Truthout*, 4 April, https://truthout.org/articles/the-covid-19-pandemic-is-exposing-the-plague-of-neoliberalism/ Accessed 7 August, 2020.

Green, Michael and Evan S. Medeiros. 2020. 'The Pandemic Won't Make China the World's Leader: Few Countries Are Buying the Model or the Message from Beijing', *Foreign Affairs*, 15 April. www.foreignaffairs.com/articles/united-states/2020-04-15/pandemic-wont-make-china-worlds-leader Accessed 1 May, 2020.

Grindle, Merilee S. 2004. 'Good Enough Governance: Poverty Reduction and Reform in Developing Countries', *Governance: An International Journal of Policy, Administration and Institutions*, 17, 525–548.

Grindle, Merilee S. 2010. 'Good Governance: The Inflation of an Idea', *CID Faculty Working Paper No. 202*, October, John F. Kennedy School of Government, Harvard University, 1–20.

Grindle, Merilee S. 2011. 'Good Enough Governance Revisited', *Development Policy Review*, 29(1), s199–s221.

Grindle, Merilee S. 2017. 'Good Governance, R.I.P.: A Critique and an Alternative', *Governance: An International Journal of Policy, Administration, and Institutions*, 30(1), 17–22.

Grovogui, Siba N'Zatioula. 2001. 'Come to Africa: A Hermeneutic of Race in International Theory', *Alternatives*, 26(4), 425–448.

Guadagno, Lorenzo. 2020. *Migrants and the COVID-19 Pandemic: An Initial Analysis*, Geneva: International Organization for Migration.

Gupta, Sunetra. 2020. 'We Cannot Look at This Epidemic as a Single Axis of How Many People are Going to Become infected', *The Times of India*, Kolkata, 3 July, 12.

Guy Peters, B. 2012. 'Governance as Political Theory', in David Levy-Faur ed., *The Oxford Handbook of Governance*, Oxford: Oxford University Press, 19–32.

Hafner, Marco, Erez Yerushalmi, Clement Fays, Eliane Dufresne and Christian van Stolk. 2020. *COVID-19 and the Cost of Vaccine Nationalism*, Santa Monica, CA: Rand Corporation, 1–61.

Hamelink, Cees Jan. 2020. 'Do Not Abuse Science for Corona Politics', 7 May, https://www.other-news.info/2020/05/do-not-abuse-science-for-corona-politics/ Accessed 1 June, 2020.

Han, Byung-Chul. 2020a. *The Disappearance of Rituals: A Topology of the Present*, Translated by Daniel Steuer, Cambridge: Polity Press.

Han, Byung-Chul. 2020b. 'The Viral Emergen(e/y) and the World of Tomorrow', Translated by Richard James Bowling, *Pianola Con Libre Albedrio*, 29 March, https://pianolaconalbedrio.wordpress.com/2020/03/29/the-viral-emergence-y-and-the-world-of-tomorrow-byun-chul-han/ Accessed 1 May, 2020.

Hannah, Matthew G., Jan Simon Hutta and Christoph Schemann. 2020. 'Thinking through Covid-19 Responses with Foucault – An Initial Overview', *Antipode Online*, 5 May, https://antipodeonline.org/2020/05/05/thinking-through-covid-19-responses-with-foucault/ Accessed 8 June, 2020.

Happe, Kelly E., Jenell Johnson and Marina Levina eds. 2018. *Biocitizenship: The Politics of Bodies, Governance, and Power*, New York: New York University Press.

Hardt, Michael and Antonio Negri. 2009. *Empire*. Cambridge, MA: Harvard University Press.

Harris, Tristan. 2020. 'A 15-year Old Influencer can Now Reach as Many People as a Newspaper but with None of the Responsibility', *Sunday Times of India* (Kolkata), 11 October, p.11.

Heath, Robert L. and H. Dan O'Hair. 2009. *Handbook of Risk and Crisis Communication*, New York and Oxford: Routledge.

Heath, Robert L. 2018. 'How Fully Functioning Is Communication Engagement If Society Does Not Benefit?' in Kim. A. Johnston and Maureen Taylor eds., *The Handbook of Communication Engagement*, New Jersey: Wiley Blackwell, 33–47.

Herman, Jonathan D. and Emily Oster, 2020. 'What We Know—and Really Don't Know—About the Future of COVID-19 Vaccines', *Future Tense*, 22 June. https://slate.com/technology/2020/06/covid-vaccine-candidates-knowns-unknowns.html Accessed 2 October, 2020.

Hernández, Javier C. 2020. 'China Spins Coronavirus Crisis, Hailing Itself as a Global Leader', *The New York Times*, 28 February. https://www.nytimes.com/2020/02/28/world/asia/china-coronavirus-response-propaganda.html Accessed 8 June, 2020.

Heydarian, Richard Javad. 2020. 'Calls Rising for China to Pay Pandemic Reparations', *Asia Times*, 25 April. https://asiatimes.com/2020/04/calls-rising-for-china-to-pay-pandemic-reparations/ Accessed 7 July, 2020.

Honingsbom, Mark. 2009. 'The Historical Key Word Pandemic', *The Lancet*, 373, 1939, 6 June.

Honingsbom, Mark. 2019. *The Pandemic Century: One Hundred Years of Panic, Hysteria and Hubris*, London: Hurst & Company.

IDeaS, 2020. 'List of Known Misinformation and Disinformation Regarding Corona Virus in Social Media', https://www.cmu.edu/ideas-social-cybersecurity/research/misinformation-and-disinformation-3-20-2020.pdf Accessed 15 August, 2020.

Instagram Community Guidelines. 2020. 'Privacy and Safety Centre', https://en-gb.facebook.com/help/instagram/477434105621119 Accessed 24 September, 2020.

ISD Policy Brief. 2020. *Covid-19 Disinformation Briefing No. 1*, London: Institute of Strategic Dialogue, 27 March, 1–14.

Issak, Jim and Mina J. Hanna. 2020. 'User Data Privacy: Facebook, Cambridge Analytica, and Privacy Protection', *Computer*, 56–59. https://dl.acm.org/doi/10.1109/MC.2018.3191268 Accessed 4 October, 2020.

Jamet, Romuald. 2020. 'The Promises and Pitfalls of Algorithmic Governmentality', *Global-e*, 13, 67, https://www.21global.ucsb.edu/global-e/october-2020/promises-and-pitfalls-algorithmic-governmentality Accessed 7 October, 2020.

Jaye, Nathan. 2017. 'Interview with Michele Wucker: Do "Gray Rhinos" Pose a Greater Threat Than Black Swans?' *CFA Institute Magazine*, 23 October. https://blogs.cfainstitute.org/investor/2017/10/23/do-gray-rhinos-pose-a-greater-threat-than-black-swans/ Accessed *3 July, 2020*.

Johnston, Kim A. 2018. 'Toward a Theory of Social Engagement', in Kim. A. Johnston and Maureen Taylor eds., *The Handbook of Communication Engagement*, New Jersey: Wiley Blackwell, 19–32.

Jolley, Rachael. 2020. 'Editorial: A Question of Trust: It's Hazardous to Discourage Thought, and to Undermine Trust, Especially in a Crisis', *Index on Censorship*, 41(2), 1–3.

Jones, Branwen Gruffydd. 2013. 'Good Governance' and 'State Failure': Genealogies of Imperial Discourse', *Cambridge Review of International Affairs*, 26(1), 49–70.

Kang, Cecilia and Mike Isaac. 2020. "U.S. and States Say Facebook Illegally Crushed Competition", *The New York Times*, 9 December.

Khoo, Su-ming. 2020. 'COVID-19 Pandemic Ignorance and the 'Worlds' of Development', in Pádraig Carmody, Gerard McCann, Clodagh Colleran, Ciara O'Halloran eds., *COVID-19the Global South: Impacts and Responses*, Bristol: Bristol University Press, 7–16.

Kindig, Jessie, Mark Krotov and Marco Roth. 2020. *There Is No Outside: COVID-19 Dispatches*, London: n+1 &Verso. www.versobooks.com/books/3620-there-is-no-outside Accessed 6 June, 2020.

Klein, Naomi. 2020. 'How Big Tech Plans to Profit from the Pandemic', *The Guardian*, 13 May, https://www.theguardian.com/news/2020/may/13/naomi-klein-how-big-tech-plans-to-profit-from-coronavirus-pandemic Accessed 22 October, 2020.

Kloet, Jeroen de, Jian Lin and Yiu Fai Chow. 2020. "We are Doing Better': Biopolitical Nationalism and the COVID-19 Virus in East Asia', *European Journal of Cultural Studies*, 1–6, https://journals.sagepub.com/doi/pdf/10.1177/1367549420928092 Accessed 9 August, 2020.

Klous, Sander and Nart Wielaard. 2016. *We Are Big Data: The Future of the Information Society*, Amsterdam: Atlantis Press.

Kooiman, Jan and M. Van Vliet. 1993. 'Governance and Public Management', in K. Eliassen and J. Kooiman eds., *Managing Public Organisations: Lesson from Contemporary European Experience*, London: Sage.

Krekó, Péter and Patrik Szicherle. 2020. 'Gone Viral: COVID-19 in the Disinformation Ecosystem', *Eurozine*, 17 March.

Lapavistas, Costas. 2020. 'This Crisis Has Exposed the Absurdities of Neoliberalism. That Doesn't Mean It'll Destroy It', *Jacobin*, 27 March, https://www.jacobinmag.com/2020/03/coronavirus-pandemic-great-recession-neoliberalism Accessed 15 June, 2020.

Leach, Melissa and Mariz Tadros. 2014. 'Epidemics and the Politics of Knowledge: Contested Narratives in Egypt's H1N1 Response', *Medical Anthropology: Cross-Cultural Studies in Health and Illness*, 33(3), 240–254.

Leaders. 2020. 'COVID-19 is Here to Stay. People Will Have to Adopt'. *The Economist*, 4 July. https://www.economist.com/leaders/2020/07/04/covid-19-is-here-to-stay-people-will-have-to-adapt?fsrc=newsletter&utm_campaign=the-economisttoday&utm_medium=newsletter&utm_source=salesforce-marketing-cloud&utm_term=2020-07-03&utm_content=article-link-1 Accessed 4 July, 2020.

Lemke, Thomas. 2011. *Biopolitics: An Advanced Introduction*, Translated by Eric Frederick Trump, New York and London: New York University Press.

Lent, Jeremy. 2020. 'Coronavirus Spells the End of the Neoliberal Era. What's Next?' *Patterns of Meaning*, 2 April, https://patternsofmeaning.com/2020/04/02/coronavirus-spells-the-end-of-the-neoliberal-era-whats-next/ Accessed 19 June, 2020.

Levitt, Michael. 2020. 'The Nobel Prize-Winning Scientist: The COVID-19 Epidemic was Never Exponential', *The Post*, 2 May. https://unherd.com/thepost/nobel-prize-winning-scientist-the-covid-19-epidemic-was-never-exponential/ Accessed 4 July.

Levy-Faur, David. 2012. 'From "Big Government" to "Big Governance"', in David Levy-Faur ed., *The Oxford Handbook of Governance*, Oxford: Oxford University Press, 3–18.

Li, Heidi Oi-Yee, Adrian Bailey, David Huynh and James Chan. 2020. 'YouTube as a Source of Information on COVID-19: A Pandemic of Misinformation?', *BMJ Global Health*, Aprill, 1–6.

Liesen, Laurette T. and Mary Barbara Walsh. 2012. 'The Competing Meanings of "Biopolitics" in Political Science: Biological and Postmodern Approaches to Politics', *Politics and the Life Sciences*, 31(1/2), 2–15.

London, Alex John and Jonathan Kimmelman. 2020. 'Against Pandemic Research Exceptionalism', *Science*, 368(6490), 476–477.

Lorenzini, Danielle. 2020. 'Biopolitics in the Time of Coronavirus', *Critical Inquiry*, 2 April, https://critinq.wordpress.com/2020/04/02/biopolitics-in-the-time-of-coronavirus/ Accessed 31 July, 2020.

Lowi Institute. 2021. https://interactives.lowyinstitute.org/features/covid-performance/ 13 March Accessed 7 April, 2021.

Lupton, Deborah and Karen Willis eds. 2021. *The COVID-19 Crisis: Social Perspectives*, London and New York: Routledge.

Lyotard, Jean-François. 1984. *The Postmodern Condition: A Report on Knowledge*, Minneapolis: Minnesota University Press.

Makridakisa, Spyros, Robin M. Hogarthb and Anil Gaba. 2009. 'Forecasting and Uncertainty in the Economic and Business World', *International Journal of Forecasting*, 25, 794–812.

Manski, Charles F. 2020. '*Coping with COVID Uncertainties*', *Paper presented at the Third IESR-GLO Joint Conference*, June. https://faculty.wcas.northwestern.edu/~cfm754/covid_uncertainties.pdf Accessed 13 July, 2020.

Manski, Charles F. 2020b. 'COVID-19 Policy Must Take All Impacts into Account', *Scientific American*, 28 March, https://www.scientificamerican.com/author/charles-f-manski/ Accessed 15 April, 2020.

Mansnerus, Erika. 2010. 'Silence of Evidence in the Case of Pandemic Influenza Risk Assessment', Centre for Analysis of Risk and Regulation, London School of Economics and Political Science, Discussion Paper No. 60, February, 1–17.

Marshall, T.H. 1992. 'Citizenship and Social Class', in T.H. Marshall and Tom Bottomore eds., *Citizenship and Social Class*, London: Pluto Press, 8–17. The essay was originally published in 1950.

Marx, Karl. 1843. *Critique of Hegel's Philosophy of Right*. www.marxists.org/archive/marx/works/1843/critique-hpr/ch03.htm Accessed 18 July, 2020.

Mazzucato, Mariana. 2020. 'The Covid-19 Crisis is a Chance to do Capitalism Differently', *The Guardian*, 18 March, https://www.theguardian.com/commentisfree/2020/mar/18/the-covid-19-crisis-is-a-chance-to-do-capitalism-differently Accessed 8 April, 2020.

Mbembe, Achille. 2003. 'Necropolitics', *Public Culture*, 15(1), 11–40.

Mbembe, Achille. 2020. 'The Pandemic Democratizes the Power to Kill. An Interview', *European Journal of Psychoanalysis*, 13(1), https://www.journal-psychoanalysis.eu/the-pandemic-democratizes-the-power-to-kill-an-interview/ Accessed 24 October, 2020.

McMillen, Christian W. 2016. *Pandemics: A Very Short Introduction*, New York: Oxford University Press.

Medley, Graham. 2020. 'Interview: Coronavirus: Can Herd Immunity Protect the Population?' 13 March, www.bbc.co.uk/programmes/p086hjgc Accessed 14 April, 2020.

Meikle, Graham. 2016. *Social Media: Communication, Sharing, and Visibility*, New York: Routledge.

Mirowski, Philip. 2013. *Never Let a Serious Crisis Go to Waste: How Neoliberalism Survived the Financial Meltdown*, London and New York: Verso.

Mitchell, Katharyne. 2016. 'Neoliberalism and Citizenship', in Simon Springer, Kean Birch and Julie MacLeavy eds., *The Handbook of Neoliberalism*, London and New York: Routledge, 118–129.

Morens, David M., Gregory K. Folkers, and Anthony S. Fauci. 2009. 'What is a Pandemic?' *The Journal of Infectious Diseases*, 200(7), 1018–1021.

Naidoo, Kiasha. 2020. 'How COVID-19 Reveals the Paradoxes of Neoliberal Logic', *Elephant*, 9 May, https://www.theelephant.info/op-eds/2020/05/09/how-covid-19-reveals-the-paradoxes-of-neoliberal-logic/ Accessed 2 August, 2020.

Nancy, Jean-Luc. 2020. 'Eccezione Virale', *Antinomie*, 27 February. www. antinomie.it/index.php/2020/02/27/eccezione-virale/I have used the English version, 'Coronavirus and Philosophers: Jean-Luc Nancy--- Viral Exception', *European Journal of Psychoanalysis*, www.journal-psychoanalysis.eu/coronavirus-and-philosophers/ Accessed 1 July, 2020.

Negri, Antonio. 1989. *The Politics of Subversion: A Manifesto for the Twenty-First Century*, Translated by James Newell, Cambridge: Polity Press.

Newman, Janet. 2001. *Modernizing Governance: New Labour, Policy and Society*, London: Sage.

News. 2020. 'WHO Chief Chastises World Leaders for 'Mixed Messages'', *The Times of India*, 15 July, 13.

Nixon, Kari and Lorenzo Servitje eds. 2016. *Endemic: Essays in Contagion Theory*, London: Palgrave Macmillan.

Olsen, Niklas and Daniel Zamora. 2020. 'Pandemics Show How the Free Market Fails Us', *Jacobin*, 26 March, www.jacobinmag.com/2020/03/coronavirus-covid-19-capitalism-free-market-crisis Accessed 17 July, 2020.

O'Neil, Cathy. 2016. *Weapons of Math Destruction: How Big Data Increases Inequality and Threatens Democracy*, New York: Crown Publishers.

Oxford Reference. 2017. *Oxford Essential Quotations*, ed. Susan Ratcliffe. Oxford: Oxford University Press. www.oxfordreference.com/view/10.1093/acref/9780191843730.001.0001/q-oro-ed5-00008992 Accessed 3 January, 2020.

Paho-WHO Factsheet. 2020. 'Understanding the Infodemic and Misinformation in the Fight against COVID-19, PAHO/IMS/EIH/COVID-19/20-0006', *Pan American Health Organization*, 1–4.

Pandemic Response Report. 2009. 'Pandemic Response Governance Framework', *Government of Alberta*, 1–24.

Parry, Bronwyn. 2012. 'Domesticating Biosurveillance: 'Containment' and the Politics of Bioinformation', *Healthplace*, 18(4), 718–725.

Peters, Michael A. 2012. 'Bio-informational Capitalism, *Thesis Eleven*, 110(1), 98–111.

Peters, Michael A. 2020. 'Love and Social Distancing in the Time of Covid-19: The Philosophy and Literature of Pandemics', *Educational Philosophy and Theory*, 53(8), 1–5.

Peters, Michael A., Petar Jandrić and Peter McLaren. 2020. 'Viral Modernity? Epidemics, Infodemics, and the 'Bioinformational' Paradigm', *Educational Philosophy and Theory*, 1–23. https://www.tandfonline.com/doi/pdf/10.1080/00131857.2020.1744226

Pierre, J. and G. Stoker. 2000. 'Toward Multilevel Governance', in P. Dunleavy, A. Gamble, I. Holliday, and G. Peele eds., *Developments in British Politics 6*, London: Palgrave Macmillan, 29–44.

Plows, Alexandra and Paula Boddington. 2006. 'Troubles with Biocitizenship?' *Genomics, Society and Policy*, 2(3), 115–135.

Posetti, Julie and Kalina Bontcheva. 2020. *Disinfodemic: Deciphering the COVID-19 Disinformation*, Paris: UNESCO-International Society for Journalists, https://en.unesco.org/covid19/disinfodemic/brief1 Accessed 29 September, 2020.

Prashad, Vijay. 2020. 'A Socialist Cry for Civilisational Change: COVID-19 and the Failure of Neo-liberalism', *Economic and Political Weekly*, 55(16), 18 April, https://www.epw.in/engage/article/socialist-cry-civilisational-change-covid-19-coronavirus Accessed 1 May, 2020.

Qiu, W. S. Rutherford, A. Mao, and C. Chu. 2016–2017. 'The Pandemic and its Impacts', *Health, Culture and Society*, 9/10, 1–11.

Rainbow, Paul and Nikolas Rose. 2006. 'Biopower Today', *Biosocieties*, 1(2), 195–217.

Rainbow, Paul and Nikolas Rose. n.d. 'Thoughts on the Concept of Biopower Today', http://ayp.unia.es/dmdocuments/umbrales15.pdf Accessed 4 August, 2020.

Ramji-Nogales, Jaya and Iris Goldner Lang. 2020. 'Freedom of Movement, Migration, and Borders', *Journal of Human Rights*, 19(5), 593–602.

Reed, Jason. 2020. 'I'm a Conservative Neoliberal—But Right Now, the State Needs to Spend Big on Helping People', *Prospect*, 20 March. https://www.prospectmagazine.co.uk/politics/coronavirus-ubi-funding-grants-businesses-uk-boris-johnson Accessed 1 April, 2020.

Report 1. 2020. *Report of the WHO-China Mission on Coronavirus Disease 2019 (COVID-19)*. 16–24 February, 1–40. Publisher and place of publication not mentioned.

Repucci, Sarah and Amy Slipowitz. 2020. *Democracy under Lockdown: The Impact of COVID-19 on the Global Struggle for Freedom*, Washington: Freedom House, 1–17.

Reynolds, Lindsey and Salla Sariola. 2018. 'The Ethics and Politics of Community Engagement in Global Health Research', *Critical Public Health*, 28(3), 257–268.

Reynolds, Lindsey and Salla Sariolla. 2020. *The Ethics and Politics of Community Engagement in Global Health Research*, London and New York: Routledge.

Rhodes, R. 1996. 'The New Governance: Governing without Government', *Political Studies*, 44, 652–667.

Roberts, Stephen L. and Stefan Elbe. 2016. 'Catching the Flu: Syndromic Surveillance, Algorithmic Governmentality and Global Health Security', *Security Dialogue*, 48(1), 1–17.

Rodrik, Dani. 2020. 'Will COVID-19 Remake the World?' *Project Syndicate*, 6 April. www.project-syndicate.org/commentary/will-covid19-remake-the-world-by-dani-rodrik-2020-04?barrier=accesspaylog Accessed 12 July, 2020.

Roe, Emery. 2020. 'Control, Manage or Cope?: A Politics for Risks, Uncertainties and Unknown-Unknowns', in Ian Scoones and Andy Sterling eds., *The Politics of Uncertainty: Changes of Transformation*, London and New York: Routledge, 73–84.

Rory, Smith, Seb Cubbon and Claire Wardle. 2020. 'Under the Surface: COVID-19 Vaccine Narratives, Misinformation and Data Deficits on Social Media', 1–96, https://firstdraft-news.org/vaccinenarratives-full-report-november-2020 Accessed 11 December, 2020.

Rose, Nikolas and Carlos Novas. 2004. 'Biological Citizenship', in Aihwa Ong and Stephen J. Collier eds., *In Global Assemblages: Technology, Politics, and Ethics as Anthropological Problems*, London: Blackwell, 439–463.

Saad-Filho, Alfredo. 2020. 'Coronavirus, Crisis, and the End of Neoliberalism', *Socialist Project: The Bullet*, 17 April, https://socialistproject.ca/2020/04/coronavirus-crisis-and-the-end-of-neoliberalism/#more

Sarasin, Philipp. 2020. 'Understanding the Coronavirus Pandemic with Foucault?' www.fsw.uzh.ch/foucaultblog/essays/254/understanding-corona-with-foucault Accessed 2 August, 2020.

Sastry, Shaunak and Mohan J. Dutta. 2017. 'Health Communication in the Time of Ebola: A Culture-Centered Interrogation', *Journal of Health Communication*, 22, 10–14.

Saulnier, Alana. 2017. 'Surveillance as Communicating Relational Messages: Advancing Understandings of the Surveilled Subject', *Surveillance & Society*, 15(2), 286–302.

Schrecker, Ted and Claire Bramba. 2015. *How Politics Makes Us Sick: Neoliberal Epidemics*, Hampshire: Palgrave Macmillan.

Schubert, Kirsten. 2020. 'Crying for Repression: Populist and Democratic Biopolitics in Times of COVID-19', *Critical Legal Thinking*, 1 April, https://criticallegalthinking.com/2020/04/01/crying-for-repression-populist-and-democratic-biopolitics-in-times-of-covid-19/ Accessed 28 July, 2020.

Seaton, Jean, Amy Sippet and Ben Worthy. 2020. 'Fact Checking and Information in the Age of Covid', *Political Quarterly*, 91(3), July–September, 578–584.

Seidel, G. and L. Vidal. 1997. 'The Implications of 'Medical', 'Gender in Development' and 'Culturalist' Discourses for HIV/AIDS Policy in Africa', in C. Shore and S. Wright ed., *Anthropology of Policy: Critical Perspectives on Governance and Power*, London and New York: Routledge, 59–87.

Sellnow, Timothy L. and Matthew W. Seeger. 2013. *Theorizing Crisis Communication*, Malden, MA: Wiley-Blackwell.

Shepherd, Gregory J. and Eric W. Rothenbuhler. 2013. *Communication and Community*, New York and London: Routledge.

Shermer, Michael. 2005. 'Rumsfeld's Vision: Where the Known Meets the Unknown is Where Science Begins', *Scientific American*, 1 September, https://www.scientificamerican.com/article/rumsfelds-wisdom/ Accessed 3 January, 2020.

Sinha, Dipankar. 2018. *The Information Game in Democracy*, London and New York: Routledge.

Sinha, Dipankar. 2021a. *The Social Sciences in a Global Age: Decoding Knowledge Politics*, London and New York: Routledge.

Sinha, Dipankar. 2021b. 'Public Policy Communication: Reclaiming a 'Nearly Lost Theme'', in Rumki Basu ed., *Democracy and Public Policy in the Post-COVID-19 World: Choices and Outcomes*, London and New York: Routledge, 47–59.

Sinha, Disha. 2021. 'What Are Trending AI-based Research Ideas in this Current Scenario?' *Analytics Insight*, 30 April, https://www.analyticsinsight.net/what-are-trending-ai-based-research-ideas-in-this-current-scenario/ Accessed 1 May, 2021.

Smith, James A. and Jenni Judd. 2020. 'COVID-19: Vulnerability and the Power of Privilege in a Pandemic', *Health Promotion Journal*, 31(2), 158–160.

Sørensen, Eva and Jacob Torfing. 2018. 'Governance on a Bumpy Road from Enfant Terrible to Mature Paradigm', *Critical Policy Studies*, 12(3), 350–359.

Sotiris, Panagiotis. 2020. 'Against Agamben: Is a Democratic Biopolitics Possible?' *Critical Legal Thinking*, 14 March, https://criticallegalthinking.com/2020/03/14/against-agambenis-a-democratic-biopolitics-possible/ Accessed 17 April, 2020.

Spurk, Jan. 2020. 'The World Before and After the Coronavirus', *global-e*, 9 June. https://www.21global.ucsb.edu/global-e/june-2020/world-and-after-corona-crisis Accessed 8 July, 2020.

Standing, G. 2011. *The Precariat: The New Dangerous Class*, London: Bloomsbury.

Stefan Elbe. 2018. *Pandemics, Pills, and Politics: Governing Global Health Security*, Baltimore: Johns Hopkins University Press.

Stoker, Gerry. 1998. 'Governance as Theory: Five Propositions', *International Social Science Journal*, 50, 17–28.

Stolworthy, Jacob. 2020. 'Coronavirus: Yes Minister Scene Predicted Boris Johnson's Reaction to Pandemic', https://www.independent.co.uk/arts-entertainment/tv/news/coronavirus-pandemic-yes-minister-boris-johnson-uk-testing-outbreak-symptoms-a9396511.html Accessed 15 December, 2020.

Taleb, Nassim Nicholas. 2001. *Fooled by 'Randomness: The Hidden Role of Chance in the Markets and in Life*, New York: Texere.

Taleb, Nassim Nicholas. 2010. *The Black Swan: The Impact of the Highly Improbable*, New York: Random House.

The Community Initiative Network. 2020. 'The Community Engagement in the Context of Social Distancing', https://www.comminit.com/global/content/community-engagement-context-social-distancing Accessed 15 December, 2020.

The Economist. 2020. 'Why is Europe So Riddled with Vaccine Scepticism?' 12 December, https://www.economist.com/europe/2020/12/12/why-is-europe-so-riddled-with-vaccine-scepticism Accessed 12 December, 2020.

The Indian Express. 2020. 'If Covid Vaccine Turns you into a Crocodile: Brazilian President's Remarks Trigger Memes', 21 December, https://indianexpress.com/article/trending/trending-globally/brazil-president-bolsonaro-covid-vaccine-can-turn-people-into-crocodiles-reactions-jacare-memes-7111095/ Accessed 15 December, 2020.

The Logical Indian. 2020. 'Fact Check: Research in Italy Finds COVID-19 Is Caused by Bacteria and can be Treated with Aspirin', https://thelogicalindian.com/fact-check/italy-covid-19-coronavirus-bacteria-aspirin-21655 Accessed 8 July, 2020.

The Royal Society. 2020.'COVID-19Vaccine Deployment: Behaviour, Ethics, Misinformation and Policy Strategies', https://royalsociety.org/-/media/policy/projects/set-c/set-c-vaccine-deployment.pdf Accessed 12 December, 2020.

Thiessen, Berth. 2015. 'Conceptualizing the 'Failed State': The Construction of the Failed State Discourse', *University of Saskatchewan Undergraduate Research Journal*, 1(2), 129–139.

Thompson, Sheena. 2020. 'Social Distancing — The Communications and Compliance Challenge', *Enterprise Risk*, https://enterpriseriskmag.com/social-distancing-the-communications-and-compliance-challenge/ Accessed 15 December, 2020.

Tooz, Adam. 2020. 'The Sociologist Who Could Save Us from Coronavirus', *Foreign Policy*, 1 August, https://foreignpolicy.com/2020/08/01/the-sociologist-who-could-save-us-from-coronavirus/ Accessed 5 November, 2020.

Trummer, Ursula. 2020. 'European Borders, COVID-19, and the Economy of Home Care', *Global-e*, 13(57), https://www.21global.ucsb.edu/global-e/august-2020/european-borders-covid-19-and-economy-home-care Accessed 26 August, 2020.

UHC Report. 2020. 'Sound the Alarm - People Left behind in Decision-making on COVID',6 May, www.uhc2030.org/blog-news-events/uhc2030-blog/sound-the-alarm-people-left-behind-in-decision-making-on-covid-19-555355/ Accessed 23 July, 2020.

UNESCO Issue Brief I. 2020. *Journalism, Press Freedom and COVID-19*, Paris: UNESCO, 1–17.

United Nations Document. 2020. 'Disease Pandemics and the Freedom of Opinion and Expression', A/HRC/44/49, www.ohchr.org/EN/Issues/FreedomOpinion/Pages/ReportDiseasePandemics.aspx Accessed 19 November, 2020.

Virilio, Paul. 2005. *The City of Panic, Translated by Julie Rose*, Oxford and New York: Berg.

Wald, Priscila. 2008. *Contagious Cultures, Carriers, and the Outbreak Narrative*, Durham and London: Duke University Press.

Waltner-Toews, David et al. 2020. 'Post-Normal Pandemics: Why COVID-19 Requires a New Approach to Science', *Discover Society*, 25 March. https://discoversociety.org/2020/03/27/post-normal-pandemics-why-covid-19-requires-a-new-approach-to-science/ Accessed 9 May, 2020.

Waterson, Jim. 2018. 'Five Things We Learned from Mark Zuckerberg's European Parliament Appearance', *The Guardian*, 22 May. https://www.theguardian.com/technology/2018/may/22/five-things-we-learned-from-mark-zuckerbergs-european-parliament-appearance Accessed 3 January, 2020.

WHO Report I. 2000. *The World Health Report 2000*, Geneva: World Health Organization.

WHO Report II. 2017. 'WHO Community Engagement Framework for Quality, People-centred and Resilient Health Services', No. WHO/HIS/SDS/2017.15, Geneva: World Health Organization.

WHO Report III. 2020. 'Munich Security Conference', 15 February. https://www.who.int/dg/speeches/detail/munich-security-conference Accessed 19 September, 2020.

WHO Report IV. 2020 Immunizing the Public against Misinformation, 25 August, https://www.who.int/news-room/feature-stories/detail/immunizing-the-public-against-misinformation Accessed 19 September, 2020.

WHO Website 1. 2010. 'What is a Pandemic', www.who.int/csr/disease/swineflu/frequently_asked_questions/pandemic/en/24February Accessed 30 June, 2020.

Williams, Bernard. 2002. *Truth and Truthfulness*, Princeton and Oxford: Princeton University Press.

World Bank Brief. 2020. 'COVID-19 Crisis through a Migration Lens', Migration and *Development Brief 32*, Place of publication not mentioned: World Bank-KNOMAD, 1–37.

World Migration Report. 2020. Geneva: International Organization for Migration, 1–477.

Wucker, Michele. 2016. *The Gray Rhino: How to Recognize and Act on the Obvious Dangers We Ignore*, New York: St. Martin's Press.

Young, Iris Marion. 1986. 'The Ideal of Community and the Politics of Difference', *Social Theory and Practice*, 12(1), 1–26.

Young, Jock. 2007. *The Vertigo of Late Modernity*, London: Sage.

Zacher, Mark W. and Tania J. Keefe. 2008. *The Politics of Global Health Governance: United by Contagion*, New York: Palgrave Macmillan.

Žižek, Slavoj. 2006. 'Philosophy, the "Unknown Knowns," and the Public Use of Reason', *Topoi*, 25, 137–142.

Žižek, Slavoj. 2020a. *Pandemic! COVID-19 Shakes the World*, New York and London: OR Books.

Žižek, Slavoj. 2020b. *Pandemic2: Chronicle of a Time Lost*, New York and London: OR Books.

INDEX

Page numbers followed by 'n' refers to notes numbers